SHUT UP *and*

Keep Taking The Pills

Hazel Amanda Jones

First published 2023
Copyright © Hazel Amanda Jones
All rights reserved
ISBN: 978-1-7395665-0-0

A CiP catalogue record for this book is available from the British Library.

Disclaimer
All names and some of the details in this account have been changed in order to protect the identities of any persons living or dead. This book aims to be an honest version of events as I experienced them.

PREFACE

I earnestly wanted to be a Psychiatric Nurse. I thought it was about listening to people; sharing their pain; helping them find answers to help themselves. I discovered it was the opposite. Silencing them.

Ultimately, I was silenced by a psychiatrist who engineered my constructive dismissal when I spoke out in defence of a suicidal patient.

Meet the patients I met along the way. You'll have encountered some of them yourselves. They're ordinary people beset by extraordinary life problems. The psychiatrist in question later came under scrutiny when he (wrongly) discharged a patient who stabbed a little girl to death. He had to undergo retraining. I eventually went on to overcome many obstacles and became a counsellor.

'Shut up and keep taking the pills' is written with humour and compassion, despite the (growing) disillusionment. The strong belief that we can learn to help ourselves without taking psychoactive medication pervades the narrative, shining a beacon of light in a dark world of despair and is borne out by the many hundreds of people I've helped for the past thirty years.

LISTEN

Listen to the ones whose hearts are breaking
aching from the losses deep within
Do not enforce their silence
for the soul will fester
and the person shrivel into nothingness
bear witness to the traumas great and small
This is their time to talk

People are the experts on themselves.
We should listen to their stories.

CONTENTS

CHAPTER ONE

PRE-NURSING YEARS

The scorching sun beat down. This was good because it would dry the cement between the paving blocks. Wiping the perspiration from my brow, I stood back to admire my work. A complete herring-bone path. Can't pretend that I did all of it – just spent half the day laying the finishing bricks, but the effect was to make me swell with pride.

Two years later, whilst working as a student nurse, it was quite amusing to find that this path was outside one of the hospitals where some of the training took place. In the morning, since the day involved working with a firm of builders, I had helped take down several drainpipes from a derelict building. Herring-bone path in the afternoon. This was a far cry from nursing, so perhaps an explanation of these events may be pertinent.

In 1985, the government were trying to encourage women to return to the workplace. There was a full time six- week course running up and down the country, entitled 'Wider Opportunities for Women' (WOW). It was hoped that women who'd spent years of their lives bringing up children would find a career which gave them 'gainful employment.'

As well as providing work experience of all kinds, it helped women to practise interview skills; we were paid well to do the course; the food in the canteen was par excellence and one of the tutors was quite dishy too! My position as a student RMN had been secured some months earlier, but this was a chance to explore other possibilities to find out as best I could, if any other jobs were more appealing.

For the previous fifteen years, raising children had been the priority, although I'd had a great variety of work which fitted in with family and paid the bills. Almost anything and everything were on the agenda as long as these important criteria were fulfilled. Daddy ran away when my daughters were aged three and one respectively. For ten years, bed, breakfast and evening meals were provided for student lodgers. It was the best way to earn money, yet be at home for the children. They deserved me to be there, if they had only one parent. A means to an end. It was hard because I hated cooking, but we had a lot of adventures. Perhaps that could be the subject matter for another book!

A previous career of teacher training had been attempted but hadn't worked out, after two years of trying, because the girls were too young at aged seven and five to cope with this. Without support, another eleven years had to be waited out, with lots of jobs that fitted around them, in between, before I made yet another effort at a career, without detriment to their upbringing. It was strange on the WOW course to be back in the same building where I had pursued teacher training, fifteen years earlier. Further Education was its new purpose.

'Don't know if it's for me,' I said to my elder daughter as we walked round a vast expanse of green community space quite close to our house. By then, she was training to be a vet.

'You've enjoyed doing lots of voluntary work with MIND. Why not get paid to do it?' said my elder daughter, aiming to be supportive. This had been one of the many activities that relieved the tedium of cooking and cleaning and I'd found that yes, perhaps I did have an aptitude for it.

'Wonder if I can cope with all the demands? Shift work, reading, essays, assessments… I don't like leaving your sister, either, to manage on her own.' This was actually my main worry.

'She won't be. When you're on a late – Nanna will be there in the evening. Give her a few microwave meals and she'll be fine. I'll be back on Fridays through to Sunday evening.' Younger sister had just begun to do 'A' levels. The idea that we'd all be students together suddenly filled me with enthusiasm.

So 'Wider Opportunities for Women' helped me explore other possibilities as a way of being certain of my choice.

One of the WOW experiences was working in a Home for the Elderly. It reeked of urine in the sodden carpets. I felt terribly sorry for the residents.

Another 'taster day' was being in a bank at a counter, for the whole eight hours we were there. This latter was so mind numbingly boring that in my over eager haste to escape, I'd opened the first door I saw nearest to where we'd been 'chained' and walked into a broom cupboard!

Working with a firm of builders was not the norm, nor was it the choice of any of the other 'ladies' but the thought of open air attracted me. Being outside had led me to be a 'postie' several times in the past. So this external freedom from the classroom was as inviting, because it also took me away from the kitchen sink.

The six weeks were invaluable. There were other 'tasters' too but they all served to help me decide on nurse training by the end of the summer. Preparing for this was important. The lodgers would have to look after themselves. This was explained to them. In addition, I bought them small individual fridges (second hand). They could have use of the kitchen and of course, their rent would be substantially reduced. With this latter, as an inducement, all three of them stayed.

I took a couple of weeks off for the first time in years before starting my training. The first day would be on my fortieth birthday. It felt very fortuitous to have been accepted because the cut off age was thirty-nine.

A meeting with the WOW tutor (apt, that) was arranged, to inform him of my decision. He was slim, fragrant, and extremely funny. There was an ulterior motive for this. We had an on/off romantic relationship that lasted over two years. Bonus!

Footnote: It amuses me to think that it's taken me about five minutes or so to read out an account which spans fifteen years of my life!

*MIND is an organization of many years' standing which provides help and support for people who suffer from mental illness. Sometime later in "the wilderness years", following several jobs which were gained, lost, or left behind, I would eventually have paid work there, in 1993.

CHAPTER TWO

MORE ON BEING A STUDENT NURSE

Introductory Block consisted of six weeks' training at the end of which was an exam. Why, I wondered was the focus wholly on the physiological and biological when surely – in 'mental illness' nursing as it was called then, sometime should at least have been given to 'psychological' aspects? I passed the exam nonetheless.

Fine words were spoken about patient care. A kind of charter declared that we would strive for mutual respect; aim to understand the individual person and treat him or her holistically. 'Don't imagine you'll have the time to talk to them,' rang like a death knell to my hopes of what psychiatric nursing was actually about, as well as explaining why there was nothing about psychological thinking in the first exam we sat. Would there be more of that later?

If that idea spurred me on, I was in for growing disillusionment. 'You'll be too busy with the business of running the ward' added our tutor with a confident smirk borne of experience. Always smartly dressed in a suit, shirt and tie, his brows were perpetually furrowed.

He adjusted his local accent to command gravitas, but occasionally lost an 'aitch' here and there, when he forgot.

On one occasion, in a one to one with us students, he'd asked me why I 'appeared to be so intense' and I replied that I was probably reflecting back his demeanour. Don't think he'd considered that as a possibility. He used to be quite proud of declaring that he was 'asocial', but when he retired some years later and came back to work on the wards, he had apparently attended a course in counselling skills at the local college, to develop his empathy. It amused him that his colleagues described him as a 'hedgehog' i.e., prickly! That was our experience of him too.

There were two kinds of training at that time. You could become an SEN (State enrolled nurse) with two years' training – later phased out, or an RMN (State registered Mental Nurse) with three years' training. I was to become the latter. Further into my training I discovered it was unfortunately true. An RMN was indeed 'office bound' and rarely had time to talk to anyone.

My initial placement as a first-year student was on the most disturbed ward in the medium to long stay hospital. The other students were sent out in pairs. I was alone and very fearful. One of the main purposes of our six-week training was to ensure we were 'safe' in terms of caring for patients.

Very little was said about how we kept ourselves safe. We were taught 'Control and Restraint' for when/if a patient became violent and how to restore a good relationship with them after having hurled them to the floor! On this ward, this kind of occurrence was to be expected. Our tutor who was ex-forces referred to it as 'Muscular Christianity'!

With all that in mind, I was ill prepared for the incident which took place two weeks before the end of my twelve-week placement.

SHUT UP AND KEEP TAKING THE PILLS

Together with a Senior Staff Nurse (male), we were in a female patient's bedroom for the purpose of encouraging her to get up and get dressed. It was around 11 in the morning.

He was tall, thick set and looked as though he had the physique of someone who did weight training in his spare time.

Hilda was in her fifties, quite small and frail, but she could be obtuse and awkward at times. This was one of those times. Her voice quavered as she trembled in front of the SSN, pleading, 'No, don't, Nurse. I don't want to get up. I'm tired. I'm always tired. Plea..se. Don't make me.'

The SSN barked at her to 'Get up and Get dressed!' She refused again and lay on her bed. She had no clothes on. I moved forward to assist her but the SSN barred my way and repeated his demands, stepping towards her, menacingly. She turned onto her front and clung to her bed.

I was utterly shocked by what happened next. He swooped towards her, raked his nails down her naked back and heaved her to a standing position by one arm and one leg. She was visibly quaking; began to whimper and cry but 'became compliant.' I moved to comfort her and helped her dress. I was probably as shaken as she was. I felt sick.

For the rest of the day, I was stunned. The SSN was on a half day and went home. I spoke with a third-year student who'd befriended me. Tom had a smiley face and joked a lot, but he was kind. He'd taken me under his wing. When I asked his advice about what to do, his features became serious, concerned. The words filled me with alarm.

'No one likes a reporter.' Although he sympathised with my dilemma, he was implying that I should say nothing; that I'd somehow put myself in jeopardy.

SHUT UP AND KEEP TAKING THE PILLS

For once I had the weekend off. The Charge Nurse had taken advantage of the fact that I was a student and prior to this made me cover Christmas and New Year on the off-duty roster. I hadn't known it was customary to do one or the other but not both. The lowly status of being a first-year student on a first placement did not encourage me to feel sure about speaking out.

I wrestled with my conscience and lost a lot of sleep over that weekend, but for me there was no choice. If that was what I was expected to do, I had to speak out, or leave my training. One of our group had already left in the middle of her first placement and she was on an 'easy' ward!

On Monday morning, I approached the Charge Nurse with trepidation. I told him what I'd witnessed. Although he was small, the Charge Nurse was a heavily set man whose thick moustache scarcely concealed a face that looked permanently grim. I approached him in his office, fearing his reaction. He glowered at me. Tom's words were ringing in my ears.

'No one likes a reporter.'

The Charge Nurse said not a word but went to check the patient's scarred back which showed the evidence of what I claimed. The patient's back was all the evidence I needed.

'This is serious, Hazel. Leave it with me.'

I was relieved that he seemed to have believed me, but by no means reassured about how it would affect me.

Eventually, after much agonized waiting, a disciplinary against the SSN was convened. This took place in another part of the building where the Introductory Block had been. It was held in a long room with a long table, the length of which had to be walked to arrive before the Senior Nursing Officer and my Charge Nurse who sat facing me, together with a Union Representative, on behalf of the accused. That alone made me feel as if I were on trial, here. Everyone looked grim (but then the Charge Nurse always did). The atmosphere was tense and no one seemed to realise that it was an ordeal for me. I was on my own.

'A serious charge of assault on a female patient by SSN (named) has been brought by student nurse Hazel Jones,' read out the Charge Nurse, giving nothing away.

'We're here to examine the evidence for this, but I've examined the patient and her back shows signs of excoriation. She can't have done this herself.'

I felt more hopeful.

To begin with, a loud-mouthed nurse with ginger hair came to his defence as a character witness. 'I've worked with (she named the SSN) on several shifts, in other parts of the hospital. He's kind, caring, respectful. I've never known 'im be different. I think she – Hazel's making it up.'

I was very frightened. Feeling completely alone, inexperienced and alienated – yet I had to do it. I couldn't have lived with myself if I'd said nothing. I gave my account of what happened, following this.

The SSN was then asked for his version of events.

He stated that the patient had tried to interfere with him sexually as she bent down to tie her shoelaces.

They didn't believe him.

The Charge Nurse had at least verified that scars on the patient's back had corroborated what I claimed.

A written warning was placed on his record and he was moved to another hospital.

SHUT UP AND KEEP TAKING THE PILLS

First year students were prohibited from having their first placement on this ward in future. Not sure for whose benefit that was?

CHAPTER THREE

'PETER'

The long stay ward housed some of the most dangerous and seriously disturbed patients. It wasn't locked but risk assessments of the patients were assiduously done, almost on a daily basis. This always called for staff to be alert and aware. An eight- hour shift could sometimes feel twice as long.

The whole ward consisted of an office, a treatment room and a staff room, set side by side with a large dayroom on the other side of a corridor. Bedrooms for male patients were to the left of the corridor's end and bedrooms for the female patients, to the right.

Colours were drab; the well-trodden carpet faded, bare in some places at the front of a multitude of plastic upholstered chairs encircling the sides, where patients sat and shuffled their feet throughout the empty hours of boredom.

They were free to roam the grounds of the well-tended gardens and in some cases were even allowed to go into town, unless they were having psychotic episodes at which point, they'd be under constant observation or 'specialing' as it was known.

Most were prescribed regimes of many drugs. A few passed their time doing repetitive tasks in the IT (Industrial Therapy Department), like counting and sorting screws. Some went to Occupational Therapy which was far more pleasant. It involved painting, sewing and sometimes simple basket weaving or pottery. A few worked in the greenhouses and gardens.

Peter was in his forties. He had shoulder-length unkempt, thick black hair and a beard to match. Diagnosed with paranoid schizophrenia, he suffered psychotic episodes from time to time for which he was very heavily medicated.

Although he wasn't tall, he was solidly built. When he worked himself into a fury, he foamed at the mouth whilst threatening violence to the other patients whom he accused of seemingly imagined wrong-doing.

He had to be physically restrained on several occasions by up to three members of staff. They pinned his flailing limbs to the floor before administering a diazepam injection which calmed him and made him contrite – until next time. These episodes frightened some of the patients. Others appeared largely unmoved because they were in their own worlds of chemical restraint for most of the time.

One day, Peter began to complain long and loudly about the holes in some of his well-worn clothes. Normally, his voice was rich and deep, but when agitated, he could elevate it to a high-pitched whine. This had the desired effect of making him noticed and such was his intention on this particular day. Some patients were unkindly laughing at him for saying he had 'nothing decent to wear'.

'Why's tha bothered? Tha i'n't goin' nowhere, lad,' one of the male patients had remarked.

SHUT UP AND KEEP TAKING THE PILLS

At that, I stepped in, before the situation escalated. 'Hey, Peter. Come and show me what's wrong. Let's see if I can help.'

I discovered a rather unusual way to soothe him. I mended his clothes. Over the fourteen weeks of this placement, he brought me piles of worn garments. I obliged, by sewing up the holes and tears. Sometimes, he sat beside me, fascinated by the movements of the needle and thread.

'I love watching you do this, Hazel. It's as if the holes disappear by magic. You're so clever!'

He continually poured out his thanks in that warm, deep voice. The lines of suffering on his face seemed to disappear temporarily, along with the holes I was mending.

By the end of some shifts, my fingers were sore, but it was all worthwhile, to see the pleasure it gave him.

Another day, towards the end of my time there, I was walking down the long drive to the main road where I caught my bus. Easter was almost upon us and a two-week break was in sight for us students, as well as the end of this placement.

To my amazement, I saw a sturdy figure striding towards me. It was Peter, brandishing an enormous bunch of daffodils which he'd obviously gathered from the hospital grounds. This was not allowed!

'For you, Hazel,' he said as he thrust them into my hands. 'No one has ever done what you did for me and I'm very grateful.'

My two hands could barely span the 'bouquet' but I accepted it with a sincere and gracious, 'Thank you, Peter. That's very kind.'

He turned on his heels and strode back towards the hospital. So large was the bunch, I felt I should have bought a ticket for it. I received some very funny looks from bemused passengers!

SHUT UP AND KEEP TAKING THE PILLS

Three years later, at the end of my training, I was in charge of one of the acute wards at another hospital in a different part of town. Who should be admitted but Peter, in a state of florid psychosis?

He seemed to be reassured when he recognised me, but it wasn't long before he began to march round and round the corridors that connected the rooms. He was in a state of great agitation, muttering incoherently to himself. What made matters worse, I discovered, was that he had been availing himself of chocolate from the patients' vending machine which was located well out of view of the office. He was a Type 1 diabetic, so this bad news complicated matters, just as I was about to go off duty.

A nursing assistant was asked to 'special' him whilst I gave handover to the night staff. He featured prominently in the report.

'Don't worry,' said Aisling, who was a no- nonsense Irish nurse with many years' experience under her belt. 'I'll handle him.' The diazepam injection was the only option before he gave himself a hyperglycaemic attack. I left him in her capable hands.

The next morning, on the dayshift, a chastened and subdued Peter hovered outside the office. He obviously had something important to say. He had a confession to make, he said, head hanging low.

'Oh, Hazel. I really loved you, but I've fallen for someone else. Aisling! What a wonderful woman!'

Peter's contrite expression was so sincere, my instinct was to comfort him, as you would with a child. 'She *is* wonderful, Peter,' I said and 'I don't mind at all.'

I experienced a huge sense of relief at his words. I'm not sure what Aisling thought about her new admirer, because once again, as often happened during training, this was my last shift on this ward.

CHAPTER FOUR

UNTOLD

Her parents brought her in. Voluntary admission. Marie was
seventeen, thin and pale. She looked more like a ten-year-old. Her
clothes were not what you'd expect of a teenager. Short skirts and
short coats were all the rage. Marie's coat was unfashionably long.
A baggy jumper attempted to hide an underweight frame. Her
parents were smartly attired but mute. What was there to say? She
was 'under' the professionals now and they felt they'd done the right
thing by bringing her here. So, they didn't say anything, at least, not
when I was there.

Their address had suggested that they came from a side of town that
was reputed to be quite well to do. They seemed to be consumed by
concern. Frowning. Hovering anxiously... but did I notice that their
daughter flinched ever so slightly, almost imperceptibly when her
father attempted to put his arm round her shoulders?

I was not privy to what the parents had said, nor did I learn any
words of wisdom from the psychiatrist's intervention. We were told
in a handover, during which information was given about patients,
before staff changed shift, that she was self-harming (cutting criss-
crosses on her wrists) and hearing voices which were threatening

her, as well as telling her to perform even more injurious behaviours on herself.

Hearing voices? The psychiatrist had diagnosed schizophrenia. Inevitably, the drugs that would quieten her were prescribed and zealously administered. The Charge Nurse liked a peaceful, orderly ward. He was 'paternalistic' but could be strict and stern with a 'no nonsense' approach. The Charge Nurse had simply said, 'She's a troubled girl,' but I privately wondered if that should have been 'She's a girl in trouble?'

Patients, however, were 'zombified' before they had a chance of opening their mouths. At least, that's how I saw it. Some would say that the medication calmed and soothed them. Psychiatrists focused on the behaviours. I always wanted to know what was behind them. Bit of a race against time. Could I build the trust and enable the client to talk? Unfortunately, I had one week's holiday booked. I could be almost certain that she'd still be there when I returned but in what state of mind?

When I was next on shift, she was cowering in a small room that was reserved for private interviews. 'Handover' in which between shifts, nursing staff updated incoming staff about their charges, had not been promising. Much 'attention seeking behaviour' (often expressed with scorn) had been in evidence. What kind of 'attention seeing behaviour' was rarely specified! The use of the phrase was enough to elicit least concern from nurses and doctors alike. She was on 'Constant obs' (suicide watch). I believed 'attention seeking behaviour' was a disguised, often silent cry for help.

Even as this information was being delivered, there was a loud bang from the dayroom and screaming could be heard from some of the female patients. When we raced there, she was semi-conscious on the floor. She'd launched herself at the reinforced glass window in an attempt to kill herself. We were three floors up in the Psychiatric part of a gloomy old Victorian Hospital, the larger part of which was given over to the General side.

She was very bruised after falling back into the room onto the wooden arms of two chairs and had cut her head open on the corner of a table. These injuries necessitated a stay on the General side of the hospital, accompanied by a nurse or nurses who'd carry on the 'specialing' (another name for suicide watch). It didn't involve me because I was a student in my first year of training.

I have to mention here that this was one of three 'acute' wards which received patients who, for the most part were frantically distressed, given to self-harming behaviours and frequently on a Section 2. This meant that they could be detained up to 28 days in order to be risk assessed before deciding what their treatment should be.

Marie, however was 'voluntary', although who had volunteered her was questionable. She was limp and dejected, appearing to have no volition at all. The 'acting out' of 'paranoid behaviour' was blamed on her diagnosed illness.

Trained nurses were quite matter of fact about this. Would I respond in that way after my training? I doubted it somehow. I was viscerally shaken. Qualified staff on the other hand, seemed to accept unquestioningly, that her actions could be explained by the schizophrenia diagnosis.

When she returned, the heavy drug regime had taken hold. Her eyes were glazed, her speech monosyllabic. But she was 'compliant.' So much so, that over the weekend, it was proposed she should be allowed home leave. Before this, I'd tried to talk to her. She'd told me how worthless she felt and said that the voices were telling her to kill herself.

'I'm no good,' she kept saying, repeatedly. By then, she seemed resigned and hopeless. Sadly, I feared she was beyond counselling. Her mind was fogged by the medication.

'I don't think she should go on home leave,' I'd said at handover, towards the end of the week. 'She's very low in mood and self-esteem. I think she's at risk of harming herself. Did you see her flinch when her dad tried to put his arm round her?'

No one else had. My concerns were voted down. Trained staff thought it would do her good to go home and be in 'normal surroundings.' The psychiatrist was guided by the trained staffs' view, so my objections to this were overruled and when I wasn't on duty, she was 'let out.' I was only a first-year student after all.

I never saw her again. That weekend, she became another statistic when she hurled herself over the local railway bridge as a train was passing through.

It was her mother who came to the ward to collect her few possessions. I gave her my heartfelt condolences. She smiled sadly and said: 'My husband couldn't come. She was "Daddy's little girl." He loved her too much.'

EMOTIONAL ALCHEMY

I have held the hands of broken souls whose lives disintegrated

I have stemmed the blood from self-inflicted wounds
paced miles with those on 'constant obs'
down endless corridors
and countered suicidal arguments with gentlest persuasion.

Played useless games of draughts and dominoes
in soulless dayrooms
passing time and hoping drugs would heal their pain.

I have sought to help them regain strength
to engage in the battle of life once more
and live it to the full.

Walked with them through 'the shadowy valley'
shared grief and rage in pastel-painted rooms.
Listened to their stories, borne witness to their suffering
until they could emerge with courage and determination
find self-belief in power that would sustain them.

Helped them help themselves through tribulations
we all must face and must survive or die.

Hope is the balm and antidote for despair
Most powerful medicine of all.

CHAPTER FIVE

'ANNA-MAE'

Anna Mae's pretty, oriental features were contorted in fury when she was 'escorted' onto the ward by two male auxiliaries. Her screams of protest reverberated around the walls of the corridor. They marched her to the seclusion room 'for her own protection' and that of the other patients. Padded. Bed on the floor. Bars at the window.

'She's a regular,' observed one of the Staff Nurses, in an uncaring tone that seemed to imply she deserved little attention. This was compounded by her next utterance, laced with sarcasm, 'We'll have the pleasure of her company for the next month or more.'

Not all nurses were so dismissive, but for some, this was their way of coping. By this, I deduced that Anna-Mae had been brought in under a Section 2 of The Mental Health Act for observation and assessment and treatment, over a period of 28 days.

Relays of qualified staff would 'special' her over the next few days. Major tranquillisers would subdue her angry outbursts. In Anna Mae's case, more than one was prescribed.

She spoke very little English but had manufactured an expression of contempt by contracting two words into the expostulation 'Stupig!!!'

For some inexplicable reason, this endeared her to me. When she spat this word out, her eyes would flash and she'd turn on her heel and march away, in a gesture of defiance. Some of her frustration with staff was about not being able to make herself understood, even though she spoke broken English. Her accent impeded this.

I wanted to work with her. A newly qualified (and enlightened) Staff Nurse on this ward encouraged the use of counselling, but how to counsel someone who barely spoke the language was a hurdle. I canvassed the hospital for an interpreter. Before too long, a dental technician volunteered.

I made a verbal contract with her to understand the boundaries of confidentiality. That is, she understood that what she heard on the ward, stayed on the ward.

We used the small room that doubled as a break room for staff. It had a linoleum floor and dingy chairs. A couple of nicotine-stained pictures hung on the walls. I invited the interpreter to ask Anna-Mae, politely if she'd be willing to speak with me. Essentially, I asked her to tell me all about herself.

Progress was very slow, but what I learned was a revelation. This was Anna-Mae's fifth admission over the past two years. She had been diagnosed with paranoid schizophrenia, even though *no-one had ever actually talked to her during that time*. The psychiatrist 'knew' this from her behaviours.

That was all too often the basis for a diagnosis. They rarely gave any airspace to a patient to tell their story or imagine that what they were witnessing were normal reactions to abnormal events.

I learned through the interpreter that her background was tragic. She was hugely ashamed of the fact that her husband had another 'wife and family' two streets away from where she lived. He was verbally and emotionally abusive to her, whilst also keeping her short of money. She felt spurned and humiliated, as well as cut off and lonely. These painful emotional states were exacerbated by her impaired ability to communicate. In addition, she claimed that her husband dealt in drugs.

No wonder she was disturbed and enraged.

I was bound to report this to her psychiatrist. Of almost equal importance was the fact that the interpreter said her speech was slurred. She was over-medicated. This was fed back to the psychiatrist, too. He was kind and well-intentioned.

'Well, I'm glad you took the initiative, Hazel. It's shocking to hear of this and we must take action. I **do** think she suffers from schizophrenia, however. That really can't help.'

I was disappointed to hear that he was unwilling to do anything about the medication, but he was the expert in that department so I couldn't argue, could I?

Social workers and police became involved not long afterwards. With this kind of help, Anna-Mae's demeanour on the ward, became transformed. I heard that she'd needed no further hospital admissions during the following three years, when I was still working for the NHS.

I have to hope that she also had sustained help to withdraw from the powerful drug regime which, it had been supposed, would bring her benefit.

It has only been realised in relatively recent years that psychoactive drugs can cause worse problems for people than the so-called mental illnesses themselves.

Adverse side-effects can occur whilst taking them. Withdrawal can be even worse. Many GPs and psychiatrists do not know how to help their patients do this safely. Prolonged use of neuroleptics can ultimately bring about a state known as tardive dyskinesia. It mimics Parkinson's disease and the sufferer develops a kind of cog wheel rigidity in their limbs. Even before this there can be other physical disorders, stomach upset, sexual dysfunction, cardiac problems, to name but a few. These substances do a whole lot more than just affect the mood and can very often induce the anxiety and depression they're meant to combat! *

*Footnote: For further information about this please see an excellent book by practising psychiatrist Joanna Moncrieff entitled:

'Psychiatric drugs: the truth about how they work and how to come off them.'

For further information please see the IIPDW website (The International Institute for Psychiatric Drug Withdrawal). Its aims are to help people withdraw safely from psychiatric drugs.

CHAPTER SIX

THE PSYCHIATRISTS

Thursdays at 10.30am precisely, on a certain ward of the Acute Psychiatric Unit, heralded an event which was as predictable as it was comical.

Two long parallel corridors of the ward culminated in an open area that had two lifts. A sequence of noises – grinding as they moved up or down; swishing as the doors opened and a loud PING! to signal their completed action. Grind, swish, PING! punctuated everyday shifts with monotonous regularity.

Occasionally, there was the odd episode of great drama, accompanied by a surge of activity if a would-be escapee gained access. Restraining hands were placed on the patient in contrast to the soothing words that encouraged them back to their incarceration.

Thursdays at 10.30, Dr S would appear. His Davidoff 'Cool Water' cologne wafted through the air, preceding him as the doors opened for his entrance. For some hours afterwards, it masked the stale smells and body odours trapped in this ancient confined space.

He'd step out and stand still, so that observers could admire his carefully coiffeured silver hair, Armani suit and shoes which cost more than a nurse's weekly salary. Beaming benignly at his acolytes, some of whom drew back in awe; others of whom sniggered behind their hands, Dr S had arrived for the WARD ROUND.

His tall, stylish figure began to glide around the corridors. He had the power to free or detain patients at his will. The *DSM III had just been issued (selling out all around the world). This was the BIBLE for psychiatrists, denoting the symptoms of Mental Disorder which now boasted almost 300.

Any, or all of us, could have been included in this range, but of course it was the patients who were labelled and medicated accordingly. Whole new groups of drugs were beginning to be used which psychiatrists, I think, genuinely believed quelled if not cured the symptoms.

He stooped slightly as an old patient came scurrying down the corridor. 'Morning, my good man. And how are you today?' intoned with paternalistic enquiry and a cut-glass accent.

'Fair to middlin', Doc,' came the gruff response at which Dr S nodded, not really understanding a word of what was said. He'd admitted that he'd never fathomed the regional expressions that were uttered, but he seemed satisfied and moved on.

His status was reverentially acknowledged by many female patients and indeed some of the trained nurses. Disinhibited Dorothy was not impressed however.

When he stopped by her, she addressed him loudly in response to his polite enquiry regarding her health: 'Oo are you?' she said. 'Poncing around as though you own the place! 'Git out o' my way!' The vibrant colours of her dress and the feathered plume that flapped in her hairband, seemed in turn to add emphasis to the words she snarled at him.

Slightly ruffled, he duly did so, having had the strokes he needed for his inflated ego. He could ignore this aberration and put it down to 'her illness.'

His eager followers would then be summoned to a small room which flanked the office – therein to decide the fate of the detainees, some of whom were voluntary admissions and some of whom were sectioned.

The resulting edicts would be announced to the workforce at the next handover and with that, he executed a pirouette in front of the lift whilst it ascended to do his bidding, whereupon he would disappear until one week later.

In all my years in psychiatry, I never attended a ward round. Maybe you had to buy tickets – or perhaps be one of the chosen few. Most psychiatrists rarely talked to their patients (with one exception). They asked nursing staff about patients' symptoms, they prescribed medication, increased it, or changed it or added to it if the symptoms did not abate. Sometimes they prescribed medication to alleviate additional symptoms that were caused by the medication!

For the whole of my career as a student and then a qualified RMN, I believed and practised the idea that:

*'What we call symptoms are really a form of language waiting to find words. As soon as we are willing to go beyond the professional gaze of "signs and symptoms" we will start to open the door to the world that lies beneath it.'

This sentence is taken from a book by an enlightened psychiatrist called Dr Russell Razzaque. It epitomizes perfectly what I always tried to do. He practises in the East End of London and this book was published 32 years after I left the Psychiatric service.

*'Dialogical Psychiatry: A handbook for the teaching and practice of Open Dialogue.' Dr Russell Razzaque.

*DSM III - The Diagnostic and Statistical Manual of Psychiatric Disorders – as stated - a Bible for psychiatrists. When it came out in 1981, it outsold the actual Bible!

CHAPTER SEVEN

THE PSYCHIATRISTS - Dr A

He must have been in his late thirties when we first met, twenty years earlier. Old before his time? Although smartly dressed in a suit and matching waistcoat, his back was bent, limping with the aid of a stick, grey, thinning hair on top, yet he had a young complexion.

I learned, several years later that he suffered from a vitamin deficiency. Dr A's great attribute, however, was his kindness. He conveyed this in his voice; enunciating his words quite slowly and carefully; asking questions about what happened to patients and how they felt about it. His ability to reflect back and paraphrase what they were saying, testified to the listening skills that were fuelled by his desire to understand and help people.

Patients who wanted to see Dr A had to be prepared to wait for over an hour beyond their appointment time. His sessions were geared to their needs. He encouraged them to talk about anything and everything that worried them. There was mutual regard which fostered perpetual goodwill.

He was the only psychiatrist who visited all the wards in all the hospitals where his patients were, on Christmas Day. It was a long list which meant that his family probably saw little of him until the early evening.

Dr A believed in 'Talking Therapy' – a new and upcoming modality which had begun to be practised very rarely in the UK during the 1970s.

We may have been more than ten years behind our cousins in the US. Carl Rogers (person-centred therapist) had been Dr A's inspiration.

I (wrongly) thought that that was what Psychiatry was all about. Our student intake had the benefit of twenty hours of counselling training, during the three year course to become an RMN and this was an innovation!

Many years later, he'd greeted me warmly when I bumped into him on the Acute Unit. His face lit up with recognition.

'Hazel! How good to see you! What are you doing here?' We wore 'mufti' in this part of the hospital, so it wasn't obvious until he peered through his bottle-end glasses (eyesight was poor, too) and spotted my badge. 'So, you're training? I'm so glad to see you. I think you'll do remarkably well.'

This was an unusually brief but very encouraging encounter from a man whom I admired. He, it was, I learned after I'd qualified, had been instrumental in setting up the Counselling Department in the Outpatients' Hospital. Sadly, though at that time, the nurses who worked there had no training in counselling at all. It served simply to have an interest in that area to be involved.

The responsibility of the role was very much misunderstood – a factor which I would learn to my cost, some years further on.

Nurses and patients alike visibly brightened when Dr A entered a room.

'He's all right is Dr A,' remarked a particularly curmudgeonly inclined SEN who never had a good word to say about anybody.

Gallows humour was very much a coping mechanism that fortified staff against some of the dreadful sights and sounds that were commonplace on the acute wards, almost on a daily basis. It was part of self-preservation in an environment that was frequently pervaded with hopelessness.

Unfortunately, on the downside, Dr A was heavily into 'polypharmacy.' He seemed to welcome the new psycho-active drugs that, during that time, appeared to work miracles on the 100+ mental disorders that were listed in DSM II, (precursor to DSM III).

There was a big shift to move patients out of old institutions. So-called 'Care in the Community' was made possible by the (over) use of these drugs. People could resume independent lives in society, albeit many in sheltered accommodation. These drugs, however did not 'cure' their problems.

In the case of Anna-Mae who was Chinese and a patient of Dr A's, whom I encountered in my time as a student nurse, when an interpreter was brought in, it became clear that she had been over medicated. Slurred speech was reported – a fact that couldn't have been known without the interpreter.

Dr A, nonetheless, was a good man. He sincerely wanted to help people. After taking early retirement, perhaps as a result of his frail physical state, he bravely bore witness against one of the other psychiatrist's malpractice. Two men who were opposites of each other.

Both had the power to free or detain their charges. Dr A seemed to use his for the benefit of vulnerable people, whereas, Dr F appeared to abuse it for his own amusement. Next time, I'll write more about Dr F.

Dr A inspired me. He was the reason I came into the psychiatric profession. How did I know him twenty years earlier? He was my psychiatrist and I was his patient, at a time in my life when I had gone beyond the proverbial rock bottom.

CHAPTER EIGHT

FACT OR FICTION?

Loud exclamations were coming from the side room next to the canteen.

As I entered, the voices became subdued and sounded shocked. I landed gratefully into a shabby, well-worn armchair to eat my sandwiches. An occasional packed lunch meant I avoided time spent queuing in the canteen, which gave me additional rest for my weary feet.

Just now, however, I was more interested to learn what the nurses were clearly so excited about. Gossip was rife amongst nursing staff. It helped to pass their time, but the news being imparted on this occasion, was clearly sensational. Oblivious of me, they continued excitedly. What they said made it difficult for me to swallow my food.

'Can you really believe it?' from a plump Staff Nurse I didn't know.

All staff from all the wards converged here, so that wasn't unusual. Their cursory glances had checked out my uniform so they must have felt it was safe to continue. The Staff Nurse had clearly enjoyed the effect on her companion of the tale she had just told. It became evident she would relish repeating it. I have to say I was more than curious.

'Did you say a sabre? A real one?' The Nursing Assistant gasped as she uttered the words.

'Yes, I did,' the Staff Nurse nodded enthusiastically, but then her voice was lowered to a conspiratorial, menacing whisper, "e took it down from 'is wall, apparently and threatened to kill Dr F with it. Waved it about over his 'ead, lunging at F, in between and chased 'im out o' the house down the street!'

'Incredible!' re-joined the young nursing auxiliary who had a cherubic face, with, by now, her mouth agape.

'Oh, he's known for that sort of thing. Winds 'is patients up 'til they go mad at 'im, then sections 'em.' Her face took on an all-knowing look.

'And did 'e? Section 'im, I mean?'

'Not there and then.' The Staff Nurse gave a snort. 'He ran for 'is life as fast as 'e could, back to 'is car. But 'e went back later, mob 'anded, with the usual. GP and a social worker in tow. His word against the patient's. F had done a job on 'em. They believed 'im. Next thing you know, the poor bloke's on a section 3. 'e won't get out of that in a hurry.'

'Ow long's that for, again?'

'Six months. Detained at the psychiatrist's pleasure,' said with a degree of sarcasm.

'I didn't know they could do that.'

The Staff Nurse shrugged. She looked bemused by her companion's seeming naivete, but there was an air of resignation as well.

'He can't. 'e shouldn't. It's awful. But everyone who knows 'im knows 'e does that. 'e's not supposed to'… her voice trailed away. With a sudden expostulation, she looked at her watch and exclaimed, 'Time we weren't 'ere' and with that they arose as one and dashed off. The muttering faded into the distance down the long corridor.

The air seemed to crackle with this shocking revelation. My sandwiches lay abandoned in my lap. Could a psychiatrist really do this kind of harm? Abuse his power over people in desperate need of care? What about the Staff Nurse's observation that this was common practice for Dr F?

I was reminded of the time during my first placement when a male Staff Nurse had physically assaulted a frail, female patient in front of me. He'd raked her with his nails. A third -year male student nurse had cautioned me against saying anything, but after a weekend of soul searching, I'd felt I had no choice. I'd spoken out against the malpractice and he'd been reprimanded. A six-month written warning had been put on his record.

Yet in a later placement, I'd been dismayed to discover that word had gone round and I'd been given the label of 'A reporter.' 'We don't like reporters.' I've written about that in the next chapter.

In that moment, my heart ran cold. The options seemed to be 'put up' or 'shut up.' I knew that whatever it cost me, I couldn't do the latter. Whistle blowers had little or no protection in those times. It had only been the nail marks on the patient's back which bore witness to and verified my version of events. Otherwise, looking back now, over thirty years later, I'm fairly certain I wouldn't have had any credibility. I felt scared for the patients and scared for me.

As I moved round the different hospitals, fulfilling my placements, there were other times when staff spoke ill of Dr F. It would a further two years before I experienced first-hand, just how cruel he could be.

At another time, I'll share more of the anecdotes which circled about this man, before describing the circumstances of the encounter with him which would end my career in psychiatry.

CHAPTER NINE

TROUBLE AGAIN

'I 'ear one of you's a reporter,' said the SEN, with the unmistakeable accent of a local man; broad; flat. I later learned he was an ex-miner as were many of the male staff I encountered.

Although I didn't understand the significance of the word in this context, it startled me. A coughing fit ensued as I swallowed the wrong way.

Gimlet eyes pierced me from just below a mop of salt n' pepper curls. He affected geniality but he was arrogant and mean spirited towards patients. This manifested itself in rough handling along with chiding them impatiently.

We were on a coffee break; three of us student nurses and this SEN. No one said anything. He'd made his point. Addressing the silence now, 'No one likes reporters.'

I realised with some dismay that this remark was directed at me. Even though we were in a different hospital, several months after the event, word had got around that I'd spoken out against an SSN; been in a disciplinary. As I've said, gossip is very much part of nursing life, as it probably is in most organisations.

I felt anxiety course through my body; my palms became clammy. This bad news would have been transmitted along the 'grapevine.' I said nothing and hid my discomfort as best I could.

Two weeks later, I was assisting this SEN with the medicine round, except we were static, in the dayroom with our own captive audience, as he dispensed the drugs to them.

All the wards, corridors and dayrooms looked the same in the long stay hospital. Colourless and characterless. The beds were made of tubular iron. Their battered paint bore witness to years of use and no refurbishment. Ancient pictures that no one wanted to see, hung on the walls in a random, careless way but signifying a nod to homeliness. No fabric chairs. Faded plastic covered armchairs countered the constant incontinence of their occupants. Hard, stackable wooden chairs and formica-topped tables were brought out, to serve as a dining area during mealtimes. Functional, but cheerless.

He'd poured out a measure of Melleril (neuroleptic), when he suddenly realised that another, different drug was also needed for this patient. It had run out, so he left me standing by the drugs' trolley and marched off to the Dispensary for a replacement.

I was distracted by a frail patient, in her nineties who was deliberately hemmed in her chair by a table. She had only just been able to come off six weeks' bed rest after she'd recovered from fracturing both legs. With a degree of alacrity which belied her years, she used her thin long legs to bestride one arm of the chair in order to escape. In great alarm, I moved across the room to her, to prevent another accident. As I did so, a mobile female patient who was swifter of movement than the majority, reached out to the tumbler of Melleril and downed it in one gulp. It was not prescribed to her!

At that moment, the SEN had not returned but the Sister walked in.

I had to explain what had just happened. We were set for another disciplinary because *she* had to report it. It was common knowledge that this Sister didn't like the SEN so she pounced on a reason to have him 'cut down to size.'

A 'Shame and blame' culture was very prevalent in nursing. I often wondered why we couldn't just have a rational two-way conversation from which a better way of working could be learned and adopted thereafter.

How ironic that it was this nurse who'd said, 'No one likes reporters.'

The disciplinary (ghastly, negative word, almost implying a hanging offence) was duly convened. Again, I was a witness.

There was a simple solution. He should have put the medication in the trolley and locked it before he walked away; or preferably made certain he had all the medication that was required before he left the Dispensary in the first place.

A six-month warning was placed on his record. This was on Ash Ward. The third placement of my first year. Not surprisingly, it added to the questions I was already asking myself about whether this was *really* where I wanted to be.

In truth, I found this work to be heart-breaking. There were up to thirty people whose lives had been wrecked by different forms of dementia. Those who were in the early stages were aware of this. I felt their pain – not least because they were seeing others who had deteriorated even further. How must that have affected them? Very few had the ability to self-care. Our time was spent washing, dressing, toileting, medicating and feeding them, from one shift to the next. The medication subdued their moods. Extinguished hope? There were few visitors. Qualified staff had no time for other activities.

As a student, I had the privilege of conducting what were known as 'Reality Orientation Exercises', albeit infrequently. One such involved presenting a tray of everyday objects, then covering them over and asking the patients what they could remember having seen. It afforded some amusement to them and relieved the tedium of the hours. I also read to them as often as I could. This placement, however was one I was very glad to leave behind. Sadly, there was only one outcome for them all.

CHAPTER TEN

TO STAY OR NOT TO STAY?

The sights, smells and sounds of Oak Ward afforded a vision of the future that was too distressing to contemplate. Strong disinfectant barely disguised the unmistakable odours of double incontinence.

The patients, for the most part hobbled about in a pointless circuit from the dayroom to the bedrooms, down the single corridor that ran the length of the building and back again. A few stood by the exit from time to time, railing at their incarceration.

The door was locked for their own safety but for those who were still experiencing 'periods of lucidity' (i.e., knew what was happening), it served to remind them of their fate.

Yet more sat immobile, sad faces with unseeing expressions in their eyes, sometimes being unintelligibly noisy, often mute.

The faded multi-coloured plastic covered chairs in this dayroom were set well back to avoid accidents but placed side by side against the dingy walls. Radio 1, which seemed totally inappropriate for this elderly group of people, blared out interminable noise and inane chatter from 7am until early evening.

All students were required to experience two weeks of night shifts at this point. Nights didn't suit everyone. My permanently gaseous stomach testified to that. It was coupled with thumping headaches in the early hours.

Feelings of disorientation were compounded by the unaccustomed habit of going to sleep on the same day as later in the same day, going into work.

To fill the time overnight, I read the patients' case notes. I particularly wanted to know more about them. Perhaps this was a mistake, for so many had had distinguished roles in their lives that it emphasized and underlined the tragedy of their current condition.

A head teacher; an MP; a university lecturer; a Ward Sister. I stopped reading them because it was so distressing to think that dementia in all its ghastly forms, could condemn them to this. How much of the neuroleptic medication was used to quell their vociferous protests at suffering this fate is an unanswerable question.

Polypharmacy (use of multiple drugs) was the norm. Yet some of them must have been aware that they were expected to endure a kind of living death – surrounded by others whose brains had degenerated so much that they were reduced to the habit of playing with their own excrement; sometimes rolling it into little balls and throwing it at others.

This was another placement in my first year. I struggled with my determination to complete the course and an overwhelming desire to leave. Finding a way to make a little bit of difference was what saved me.

Mealtimes were frenzied. The patients were expected to feed themselves and a few were clearly incapable. Protracted use of neuroleptics or major tranquillisers as they were known then often cause tardive dyskinesia.

As mentioned before, this induced a kind of cog wheel rigidity in the limbs, mimicking Parkinson's Disease. They dropped their cutlery; they missed their mouths; they knocked over their drinks as they reached for them. There really weren't enough staff to help them, although some did try.

Breakfast and lunch were served on the early shift (as opposed to one meal on a late shift), so I swapped as many 'lates' as I could for 'earlies' in order to help as many people as possible have their food and drink. I saw it as a duty.

There was one patient who had the reputation of being 'a bad bugger'. Despite being quite emaciated from lack of food, Henry was strong. He was said to have 'expressive and receptive dysphasia' (couldn't talk nor understand what was said to him). I always spoke to patients as if they could understand and aimed to treat them gently, with respect.

Henry had previously managed to have very little sustenance because of impaired mobility. He was in special need of assistance which I gave him to the best of my ability, along with others who obviously struggled.

After a month or so, his relatives remarked on his improved appearance. They also seemed to be able to say that he was 'brighter'. Happier? Hard to tell when his facial features were set in a rigid stare, but he responded to me somehow with his eyes.

He was renowned for being hard to handle when being taken to the toilet.

'Never see to him on your own' said the qualified staff, but even they were amazed at how well he behaved with me.

Truth to tell, I preferred to toilet patients on my own because several of the staff 'cleaned' them peremptorily. One SEN regularly pulled a clean towel through patients' open legs after a bowel movement to avoid her having to touch them. This must have *really hurt*.

Fourteen weeks on this ward were agonizingly long. Although I gave myself a sense of purpose, perhaps achieving some small improvements, for the most part it overwhelmed me to learn and see for the first time, what life could hold for some unfortunate people. It is one of the cruellest conditions that it's possible to suffer.

The young student nurses who were my companions on this ward seemed to be completely unfazed by their surroundings. I kept the horror of it to myself. It astounded me some years later when we qualified, that five out of the seven trainees in my year, actually wanted to work in this area of nursing (Elderly Mentally Ill).

Footnote: Not long after my placement there, one of the staff was dismissed for 'cruelty'. It wasn't the nurse who practised the dirty toileting habits.

LIFE'S SORROWS

Of all life's losses – none so cruel as this
though age has withered skin, made lips too thin to kiss,
hair greyed, form stooped in painful rigid walk
the mind has robbed you of the power to talk.

Your wit and eloquence ebb away
with the relentless tide of time and every day
you lose another word, another thought
loved ones watch helpless, sad, distraught.

There's nothing that can stay its painful course
nor stem the inexorable damage from its source
your life is gone, yet living you are here
taken from you all you once held dear.

The pain's your partner's – she who sees you fall
Into the abyss. She cannot help at all.
This stage of rage and sadness will soon pass
for you – but hers is one that lasts.

Her tears are frozen deep inside with sorrow
She knows you'll fade away with each tomorrow
yet faithful she'll be with you to the end
cherishing the remnants her friend.

CHAPTER ELEVEN

A LUCKY MOVE

In the dull, paint flaked corridors that circuited the acute psychiatric ward, Mary's frail figure resembled that of a ghost. This was compounded by her pale, hollow face which became even more skeletal when she habitually sucked in her cheeks between breaths.

She was toothless. Her sparse white hair caught what little light there was as she trailed in an interminable circle.

I joined her to ask her: 'How are you, Mary?'

She took gasps mid-sentence. 'I…don't…know…what's wrong…with me.'

'Tell me how you feel.' I linked arms with her as we plodded around endless corridors.

'I don't …know…what's…wrong…with me.'

She had been diagnosed with 'agitated depression', a vague term which described but in no way explained her state. The prescribed tranquillisers and antidepressants seemed to reduce her powers of speech even further as she sank into a drug induced torpor very quickly during the course of a week.

Every time I had the chance to do so, I accompanied her on this seemingly pointless exercise, but no further information was forthcoming. We often completed our 'walks' in silence.

It would be another two years before I encountered Mary again.

Each year of the three years' training, we had fourteen days of mandatory night shifts. The second set saw me working in a medium to long stay hospital. On the acute units we wore 'mufti' as it was referred to, i.e., our own clothes, but in medium to long stay and long stay hospitals, it had to be regulation uniform. This consisted of a light blue and white checked dress, worn with a belt.

One night, when all seemed quiet, at 2a.m., the shrill, unmistakable sound of the fire bell rang long and loud. All the patients on my ward were ambulant so were evacuated very quickly. The command then came to run to the long stay section of the hospital to give assistance where it was needed.

As a Staff Nurse and I ran towards this ward, we saw a Sister appealing frantically for anyone who'd help her compete the full evacuation of her wards. Others came hurrying to wheel out bed-bound patients who were on oxygen.

'There's Mary Dawson,' shouted the Sister. 'She won't move, and I can't make her.'

On hearing a name from the past which I recognised, I asked, 'Which room? I'll go,' and darted to the far end of the corridor to find Mary.

As I entered the room, I could see Mary, clinging to her bed with a look of terror on her face, by now quite haggard and uncomprehending. I knew she might be confused by the fact that I was wearing a uniform. The last time she'd seen me, I was wearing my own clothes (on the acute unit).

'Mary. It's me. Hazel. You *know* me. I have to move you. Take you outside to make you safe.' A flash of recognition crossed her features and fortunately she offered no resistance.

It was undignified but I had to hold her under her arms and pull her backwards along the corridor for speed, gasping reassurance, every step of the way. We were the last to join assembled staff and patients on the lawn, as I lifted her over the threshold of the outer door. She whispered hoarsely, one word as I sped away to be with my group from another ward. 'Hazel.'

It had been a night of drama. Turned out it was a false alarm for which everyone was grateful.

Sometimes patients were bemused by the way that nurses 'turned up' in different areas as in our case, we changed placements. On this occasion, had it been a real fire, it would have been a blessing. A 'lucky move' because Mary let me 'rescue' her.

CHAPTER TWELVE

SHOCKS AND SURPRISES

The thought of carrying out physical tasks with patients was a disturbing prospect. The first exam we'd undertaken after Introductory Block had focused solely on anatomy and physiology.

Before he became a Registered Mental Nurse, our tutor had trained on the General Side. RGNs were regarded as 'proper nurses' compared with RMNs. I didn't share the obvious enthusiasm and special interest our tutor had for the workings of the human body. It was daunting to anticipate two weeks of attending to bodily effluents - very much akin to the aversion I'd felt when working on the EMI (Elderly Mentally Ill) unit.

It had overwhelmed me to the point where I'd considered abandoning my training. This kind of nursing was not for me. I had to prepare myself for what I feared would be a two-week ordeal.

This ward was little different from the wards on the psychiatric side. As mentioned in another chapter ('Untold'), they were all part of the same Victorian building. Gallons of magnolia paint must have been used on the walls, many years earlier. All beds were tubular iron and there were single rooms as well as four-bed 'bays'. The atmosphere was generally more cheerful than on our side, upstairs. Chemical smells pervaded the rooms but they at least gave them an air of cleanliness.

There were two surprises in store for me on this ward, however. It catered for people who'd had strokes and heart attacks. A few days in, I'd become used to the mind-numbing routine of performing 'OBS' twice daily on thirty patients. Temperature, BP, Pulse and Respirations, to be recorded on their charts; better used to the codes which regularly appeared in their notes: SOB (shortness of breath) and CPD (chronic pulmonary dysfunction) to name but two.

The nurses were a jolly bunch who joked amongst themselves and tolerated the ignorance of invading RMN students for the most part – not too many derogatory asides.

A familiar sing-song voice hailed me from one of the beds, one day. 'Hi, Hazel! Hazey May!'

This caused a sinking feeling in the pit of my stomach whilst at the same time, the blood rushed to my face. I recognized the figure of someone I'd rather not. Dark hair, partially obscuring her face, she sat, jauntily cross-legged on her bed. A number of patients who were well enough, were casting curious glances in our direction which added to my embarrassment.

With a supreme effort to be professional, I approached the bed. Sheila was a friend of yesteryear who had declared an attraction to me which I could not reciprocate.

These overtures had persisted and despite my efforts to keep the friendship, I'd eventually had to abandon contact. What could I say?

'I'm so sorry to find you here, Sheila.'

This expression of thought had something of a double

meaning.

'What happened to you?'

She'd had a heart attack, albeit mild, but was in for observations. She suffered from epileptic fits, as well, but bravely lived alone, despite her parents' protests. Although she wasn't on 'my list' which meant I had justifiable reason not to attend to her, she was difficult to avoid when she hailed me in the loudest tones she could muster.

Perhaps most disturbing was her ensuing tendency, several times daily to recount events from our former friendship in that sing- song voice, registering several decibels above the norm.

'Had a bit of a heart thing, Haze. So, it's not the old blackouts that've brought me in here, this time.'

This kind of carefree attitude to her health was the way Sheila coped with her 'petit mal' and 'grand mal' episodes.

She had better things to talk about as I soon found out!

'Hey. Haze. Do you remember when we spent hours of an evening talking about…' became almost a broadcast to the rest of the ward that was about as interesting as the shipping forecast, but a source of amusement nonetheless, if only because of the repeated anticipation.

My distress was brief, fortunately. She'd been discharged quite soon after admission, when I was off duty. I experienced a sense of relief for her because she'd been pronounced fit to go home 48 hours later – as well as relief from the uncomfortable feelings for me.

The other surprise awaited me in a side room. I saw the name first and wondered – could it be the RE tutor from the Teacher Training College I had attended? Mr S.E.J. This gentleman had had a stroke.

If people don't recover fully within 3 days of having a stroke, they are likely to be permanently impaired.

What did Mr J (for it was he) think when I appeared in his room?

He looked small and much older than I remembered him, in his hospital bed. Balding, shrunken. The stroke had taken its toll. In stark contrast to Sheila, he needed almost full assistance, being paralysed down one side – and couldn't speak.

Our relationship at college had been awkward. His remit had been to cover most of the faiths that we would encounter in schools. The keen, enquiring interest that this had engendered in me had caused me to pepper him with questions which had often confounded and confused him. I'd surmised I wasn't very likeable. He'd probably dreaded my presence.

He **was** on 'my list'. How different were the dynamics of our relationship now? I had to help him be toileted, bathed and fed when I was on shift. Once more, but for different reasons this time, I summoned my ability to be professional, aiming for kindly efficiency. To my delight, he responded. He recovered all functions, within the vital three-day period.

The question burned on my lips, so I summoned up the courage to ask him before he was discharged, 'How did you feel, when you knew it was going to be me who looked after you?'

He looked up, smiled and said, 'I was glad it was you. Glad to have someone I know who cares about how other people feel. Thank you for everything you've done for me.'

Yet again, but for different reasons, I felt a sense of relief flood through me.

I felt an even greater sense of relief when this placement came to an end.

CHAPTER THIRTEEN

THE DISPUTE

1986 saw corporal punishment banned in state schools in England, but private schools practised it until 1999. Although it was made illegal in 1986, the idea was new and not welcome in many quarters. Some Christian organizations objected to it and lobbied against it but were unsuccessful, thankfully. It was a different matter in many private households.

This placement in 1986 was with Community Psychiatric Nurses (known as CPNs for short). Student nurses were assigned to a particular nurse for the whole of the twelve weeks' duration. Between patients, 'my' CPN talked through the 'cases' we were going to see. She often came up with solutions to potential problems before we even arrived.

On this occasion, the patient was Mrs Ellis whose husband had walked out on her and their eight-year-old son, Ryan. She was said to be suffering from depression and anxiety for which she had been prescribed antidepressants and anti-anxiety drugs.

'It's the boy that's the problem' my companion muttered as we sped along the country lanes to a village far out of town. 'He's a little sod.

Drives his mother mad. She can't control him, poor woman.' The tone of her voice was soprano which somehow contrasted strangely with her large, untidy appearance. The accent was Irish, lilting. She sounded pleasant, but the words jarred.

A few minutes later, we were seated in a front room which looked as though it had been furnished from a jumble sale. The curtains were shabby, dirty and half drawn, as if defying the entrance of the sun and the outside world. There were piles of old newspapers and general junk on tables and chairs.

It had a stale, shut-in smell that spoke of its unloved state. Mrs Ellis appeared to neglect her appearance as much as her house. She had long, straggly hair which probably hadn't been washed for weeks. Her clothes were crumpled.

'I'm reet glad to see yuh,' she began. 'Ryan's been a bad un an' I gi'ed 'im a good 'iding yesterday'.

The CPN had thought better of having the cup of tea that was proffered. As if to have her theory of what constituted the cause of Mrs Ellis' diagnosis, she eagerly asked for more information about what had happened.

''e were out. 'e's allus out wi' 'is mates up to no good an' this time they'd bin throwin' stones at Mr Porter's green'ouse. Brok' t' glass, di'n't they? So I ast 'im when 'e got in, if e'd thrown any an' 'e said "no". Ah di'n't believe 'im so ah kep' askin' an' int' end e' said 'e did, so ah gev 'im wot for…'

CPN was nodding in agreement as if that were the proper course of action. Mrs Ellis went on to bemoan the fact that Ryan was 'jus' like 'is Dad; even looked like 'is Dad.'

A longer list of bad behaviours was catalogued for the benefit of justifying her punishments and the CPN by now resembled one of those toy dogs that appear on the back shelf of a car. With a spring in its neck.

There was no talk of how Mrs Ellis might cope better with her 'depression and anxiety'.

A while later in the car, I decided to say that I thought Mrs Ellis' punishment of her son was unjustified and unwise. The CPN seemed taken aback. She let out a loud gasp of disbelief.

'When he **did** tell the truth, she hit him,' I said. 'What is he going to learn from that? She should have praised him for telling the truth whilst also condemning his actions, for which, of course, there needed to be consequences and reparation. Another time, he'll learn to lie better.'

The CPN thought this was outrageous. We barely spoke on the way back to base and she avoided bidding me goodbye when the shift ended.

The next day, she had convened a meeting with the group of other CPNs who acted as a kind of jury. Their concerned faces met me as I walked into the room the following morning. I felt like some kind of outsider before anyone said anything.

'I've told my colleagues about what you said yesterday, and everyone agrees with me that Mrs Ellis did the right thing.' This was clearly not up for discussion. I kept my thoughts to myself. Her lips were pursed; her arms folded. Very much a senior putting a junior in her place.

What I **did** think was that Mrs Ellis was very angry about having been left to raise a child on her own. I also felt that she was projecting her anger onto the son who, through no fault of his, resembled his father.

Ryan was desperate to avoid his mother's wrath so frequently absented himself from home to be with his friends. She needed help with her distress. She needed help with her parenting skills. I very much doubted that antidepressants and anxiolytics would help with anything.

The sedating effects of this combination of drugs probably caused her to feel half asleep for most of her waking hours. She clearly had no energy left to look after the house, her son nor herself.

This was sadly, yet another example of how the real causes of 'anxiety and depression' were not addressed. It was believed that the medication would 'treat' the symptoms and somehow, miraculously, the patient would happily embrace life with a whole different set of feelings.

Mrs Ellis needed far more than that for her psycho-social ills, but none was forthcoming.

The CPN was utterly convinced that 'Ryan was a bad 'un' and at the root of all his mother's problems.

CHAPTER FOURTEEN

MAJOR LIFE EVENTS

At the start of my third year, I decided to move house. Lauren and Rose were both at university. It was a crazy decision. The new house had six bedrooms and there were going to be only two residents, although I had lodgers who were willing to move with me. My Mum needed support, but the house would give her the space to be separate from me as well. We weren't the best of friends at that time, so it felt safer for me, too.

I fell in love with it from the moment I walked round the rooms (thirteen in all). It was a bit unusual for a student nurse to attempt this, but I had a permanent paying job which I hoped to keep for years. How wrong I was!

The day of going to sign the papers at the building society turned out to be eventful in a way I couldn't have foreseen. It was raining just before 5 o' clock, so my future son-in-law (Rose's fiancé) Steve, drove me into town. It was touch and go that I'd get there before the building society closed. He parked in an adjoining street; I dashed out onto the road, pulling my hood up as I went, to protect myself from the downpour. I did look left, but the hood stayed put and the next thing I knew was that I was bouncing off a stationary car on the opposite side of the road; ended flat on my back, struggling for air.

Looking up at the sky, I could see worried faces peering down at me. Steve said he'd called for an ambulance at which, I raised my arm imperiously and gasped, 'Steve. *Go* to the building society!'

'I can't, Hazel. I've got to stay with you…'

I waved away his anxious looks with growing impatience, insisting, 'Steve. **Go** to the building society!' The constant repetition of this command eventually coincided with the swift arrival of an ambulance which whisked me away to hospital. I didn't know what had hit me.

Later on, with various tubes attached and an assiduous team of nurses who were constantly shining a light in my eyes, I confess that the only thing I could think about was whether or not Steve had managed to get the all-important paperwork.

The staff were annoyed when I kept raising myself up to watch the doorway. At this stage I was supposed to be lying flat on my back and not moving for twenty-four hours.

Fortunately, there wasn't long to wait. Steve and Lauren's concerned faces appeared round the door. I noted with satisfaction that he was carrying a large envelope. I reassured the nurses that I felt well, so eager was I to sign the document that would mean the wonderful house was mine.

The nursing staff reluctantly propped me up on pillows, whereupon I managed a very shaky signature on the appropriate line. Triumph!

'It was a bike that knocked you down,' said Steve, 'he accelerated when the rain pelted down at the same time as you shot across the road.' I really couldn't be bothered to talk about that, it seemed so unimportant!

We then spoke excitedly about the house. I'm sure the prospect of being in it, helped my recovery because they let me out after a couple of days.

Luckily, or so it seemed at first, I hadn't suffered any lasting ill effects.

The house move went well. It was only one street away from where I'd been living, so after several days of furious packing, by ten o'clock on the night of the move, a rather weary group of people could be seen pushing the piano along the road to its new destination. It was the final item to be accommodated in this mansion of a place.

I was so excited when we moved in, that I couldn't sleep, so at three in the morning, I got up to go and have a look around. Having only seen it once before buying it, there were so many doors - I got lost. Being space-blind and having no sense of direction didn't help.

It turned out that I hadn't escaped unscathed. About two weeks later, the dizziness set in. The GP diagnosed delayed concussion which forced me to have to stay at home for a month. At the time, this gave me a sense of great joy because I had every excuse to set about work on the house.

Lauren and Rose were there, by virtue of its coinciding with their long summer vacation. Some of their friends and mine, helped too. We had an absolutely hilarious, happy time together. We became firm favourites at the local bakery shop, from which I treated us all to sandwiches every day.

Sometimes there were up to ten eager recipients.

I suffered for this hiatus later, when my training had to be extended by the amount of time I'd had to take off, so when everyone else qualified, the number of training weeks had to be made up. I've written about the additional placement elsewhere.

The police informed me that the cyclist had thought of suing me for his damaged bike. Fortunately, they'd laughed him to scorn and dissuaded him from doing this. That would have just added insult to injury!

CHAPTER FIFTEEN

MEMORIES

Compared with the many ancient, crumbling buildings I had passed through during my placements, in training as an RMN, the Day Hospital for the Elderly was a refreshingly modern building. Light and airy, the smell of new carpets and bright paint were in contrast to the work that went on there – namely, attempts to slow down the inexorable degeneration of ageing brains. Dementia in all its forms.

Notwithstanding, the atmosphere was jolly and upbeat. Activities, throughout the day were in evidence at various tables set around the hall. All of them aimed to serve the purpose of 'Reality Orientation' which were the buzz words that described efforts to maintain the level of intellect and functioning of the participants, for as long as possible.

The 'Cognitive Function Test' which was used to assess this level, seemed to be inappropriate, at least in parts. It involved some mental maths, i.e., counting back from one hundred in sevens; remembering three words that were said, and then asking about what they were, a few minutes later.

So far, so good; but why would someone deem it necessary to be able to name the American President, nor indeed our own Prime Minister, when they were struggling to recall members of their own family? It seemed to me that the latter were more relevant and important.

At a later time in this placement, I encouraged external family members to bring in photo albums so that loved ones could be spoken of and happier times remembered. This proved to be very popular, stimulating their interest far more effectively, because it was personal.

Borrowing from ideas I'd had when raising small children and working in primary schools, I developed shopping games and games with a cardboard clock that reminded them of tasks they'd performed in the past with a sense of what mattered and when it did. This generated mutual enjoyment too. It was essentially playing, but with a purpose.

From Tuesdays through to Fridays, people attended who retained varying degrees of competence. On Mondays, we received those who were most disabled by their condition. Some could neither speak nor understand. This was referred to as expressive and receptive dysphasia.

Sylvia was someone who was said to suffer in this way. She was aged sixty, but her sparse white hair and deeply lined face made her look much older. She rarely, if ever smiled. Staff attempted to communicate with her but to no avail.

Most days, she sat by a window looking out at passers-by within the hospital grounds, rarely showing interest in anything. Staff reported that this had been happening for the past two years.

'We've tried lots of things,' said one kindly member of staff who was the life and soul of the Day Hospital. This was Edith who had been there for years.

'We've tried talking to her; we've invited her to do all sorts, but she just doesn't seem to be interested in anything. We have to assume she's OK.'

One day, I decided to try something different. I'd played 'Lexicon' (like 'Scrabble' but with cards) at a table with another patient, not far from Sylvia. Sylvia had looked over at us more than once on this occasion and it occurred to me that her facial features changed, ever so slightly. Something about her eyes. There wasn't time that day. We ended it with our usual sing-a-long of old songs which everyone seemed to love.

The following Monday, however, as soon as it was possible, I moved a table over to Sylvia's chair and dealt out the 'Lexicon' cards. She picked them up with a measure of eagerness staff hadn't witnessed in months.

Although many patients said nothing, it was vitally important to talk with them as if they understood, so I said,

'This is "Lexicon", Sylvia. You looked as though you wanted to play, last week – so here we are. Now's your chance. I'll put the first word down. Words can be built up in all directions, like a crossword puzzle.'

It was a revelation! Sylvia could not only play 'Lexicon' but she beat me consistently at every game. It was pure delight to realise that she retained this function with all the complications that the game posed.

A question was burning in my mind. Could we use the letter cards to communicate with her? The answer was 'Yes' although it was quite slow and arduous. A wonderful medium nonetheless, which might never have been discovered were it not for 'Lexicon'.

As a trainee teacher, I'd been used to creating 'flash cards' for primary school children.

On this occasion, I made additional letters out of cardboard, laminated with 'tacky back'. There weren't enough vowels and consonants in the game to be able to spell out every word, so I supplemented them. We asked simple questions with the letters and Sylvia responded in kind. That game opened up a whole new world for her and us!

Another time that stands out for me, during this placement was when I began a conversation with a very reticent patient about the fact that I had just moved house. With dementia, people can very often vividly recall their past whilst being almost unaware of the present.

She asked what the address was. When I told her, her face lit up. Pat proclaimed that she had been a servant in that house, many years ago when she had come up from the south, looking for work. (Indeed, the servants' bells were still around the house when I first moved in).

I listened in amazement as she described my house to me; the room in the attic (servants' bedrooms) which she had occupied and unmistakeably, she named the owner at that time. Pat stated that Mr B was a piano teacher. His pupils used to wait by the fire in what was a large hall at the front of the house. I had the deeds – and I knew it to be true – all of it. She'd been a teenager at the time.

Pat regaled me with fascinating stories about her life in the 1920s. Her face became animated as she recalled the daily chores of living as a house maid in what was now my house. 'We used to get up at

5am. That were 'ard, very 'ard, int' t'winter. It were so cold int 't'attic.' (I could testify to that before I had the roof insulated).

'We'd stoke up t'embers int' brick boiler int' basement. That's 'ow we 'eated t'water; then 'ad to take t'jugs up all them stairs' (39 in two flights). 'Fust fur us and then fur t'family.' It was funny how she'd almost completely lost her southern accent over the years.

There'd been a big, rather ugly partition in the hall that had screened off the kitchen from the front door. I told her I was going to have it removed.

'Oh, yus!' she said. 'It din't do for us servants to be seen by t'visitors. Family were kind, though. They treated us well. We allus 'ad a bonus at Christmas.'

In some ways this was a very sad place to work – but for me, there were moments of joy which I hope I will never forget. I haven't forgotten Sylvia and Pat and I'm still in touch with Edith.

CHAPTER SIXTEEN

A JOYOUS INTERLUDE

1988 was a year to remember – for all the right reasons, save for a bout of campylobacter enteritis which laid me low for a couple of weeks, just after I took my finals. Some weeks afterwards, the local newspaper shed light on this.

A freezer shop was prosecuted for re-freezing thawed goods caused by an electricity failure. They'd probably poisoned a lot of customers. The chicken I had opened, reeked of bacteria and this was how I became infected. I'd clapped my hand over my mouth to offset the stench and must have inadvertently transferred some of the bacteria that infected it, to me. I became very ill!

The beginning of the year, however, saw one of my happiest placements on an acute ward of mixed ages. Dr A mostly presided over these patients. I met one who would become my Best Friend a few years later and outside of work; I also met the man who would become my husband, after twenty years of living alone.

When I first saw Stella, it was to admit her to the ward. This was in the acute part of the building that was very little different from the ward to which Marie was admitted. Dayrooms, two and four bed bays flanked the gloomy twin corridors that linked them. Two lifts at one end invited would be escapees to try their luck – and they did, from time to time.

She had been brought from A&E following an overdose. Although her face was bruised and tearstained, the fighting spirit shone through her green eyes. She bristled with hostility.

'Hi, Stella. I'm Hazel. I've come to talk to you so as you can tell me a bit about yourself and we can make you as comfortable as possible.'

If looks could kill, I'd have withered on the spot from the look she shot me.

'I don't want to be here. I shouldn't be here,' she hissed.

I knew she was sectioned so I said, 'I realize that. You're here so as we know – we can be certain - that you're safe. I can see you feel angry about that.'

The force of her anger was coming towards me in waves for the next few minutes. Her fists were clenched and her face was reddening, at first. When I knew her better, later on, I think it must have been her kindness and compassion for the visible distress I was feeling which caused her to soften and talk. An exchange and gathering of information were then possible.

'I just need to take down some obvious details, Stella. Name, address, date of birth.' After this, I very gently asked, 'Do you want to tell me a little bit about how you come to be here? You've said you shouldn't be here and I can understand that.'

We had a very disturbed patient on the ward at the time and her howls and screams could be heard beyond the room in which we were talking. This must have alarmed anyone who was unused to hearing raw distress.

'Someone is very upset out there, but don't worry. There'll be a nurse to comfort her and look after her.'

My attempt to reassure Stella coincided with a quietening down of the disturbance outside.

Stella seemed to appreciate this, so then went on to describe her home life. She'd suffered the bruises from her husband. In this part of the world 'domestics' as they were referred to (fights between couples) were not uncommon, especially on Friday and Saturday nights after drinking too much. Police generally didn't intervene.

Stella had wanted to 'end it all' because she thought there was no help for her. She had suffered this kind of assault for years. I assured her many times, that what had happened was very wrong and from then on, I aimed to help her rebuild her self-confidence and self-esteem.

Finally, first 'interview' over, I asked her if there were anything I could do to help her. At that she chuckled, her face brightened and she said, 'You can get me a cup of tea!' which I duly did.

The Charge Nurse and Sister who ran this ward gave me licence to practise the kind of therapy I loved and believed in – counselling. Nine patients, out of a ward of twenty-seven, were my clients. Stella was the most receptive and intuitive of them all. We spoke regularly when I was on shift. I suggested books which she willingly read and discussed. She seemed to gain much insight from reading Anne Dickson's book, 'A woman in your own right' and Nancy Friday's 'My mother – myself.'

Her pretty face became more relaxed and happier as the days wore by. Twenty-eight in all.

When the Section Two expired, she was discharged, but whilst on the ward, her kindness and generosity of spirit extended to looking after others. In particular, she befriended Joan.

At a much later date when she was free to leave the ward, she rented the flat Joan owned. This was a mutual advantage because it provided an income for Joan and a refuge for Stella.

During this time, I did something very unconventional. With the approval of the Charge Nurse and Sister, I opted to take Joan home to live with me for a time. I'd hoped that the change of scene and a room of her own would cheer her. She was said to have 'agitated depression.'

Although she benefitted to a degree, supporting her became too much for me when, as well as full time work, I was having to study for my finals.

Reluctantly, several months on, I had to return her to the ward. Her final destination was Part III accommodation. A residential home.

When, some weeks later, I went to visit Joan, then resident at a Home for the Elderly, I feared for her welfare. She seemed to be rooted to the spot on her bed. Staff proclaimed that she rarely came out of her room. Although she had always been slim, she now looked to be the proverbial 'shadow of her former self.'

It's hard to believe it now but I sought a meeting with her consultant psychiatrist and strongly suggested *ECT. He agreed, once he'd assessed her. The home reported to me that following a course of treatment, she was a changed person.

A few months later, she visited me at home. Her shell suit (very popular in those days) was brightly coloured. It matched her mood. She announced that not only was she happy, but she had a new boyfriend!

SHUT UP AND KEEP TAKING THE PILLS

An extra placement at the end of training (written about elsewhere) had to make up for the six weeks' absence I'd had with delayed concussion, following a road accident (also written about elsewhere) but this was the ward which ultimately welcomed me as a permanent member of staff in 1989.

The patients with whom I worked discovered their strengths, added to their life skills and usually left the ward far behind, knowing that they need not return. This was one of the many joys of counselling. Helping people help themselves.

It wasn't very permanent for me, however. I lasted six months before having to have a major operation.

*ECT or Electroconvulsive Therapy is still practised in some hospitals.

The patient is sedated and electrodes are place bilaterally at the side of the head in order to give shocks which are specifically timed and counted. It's not really known how this works, but it can alleviate deep depression.

Unfortunately, it's also been linked to brain damage in some patients. This is a fact I've learned in later years and now I would most definitely not recommend it. In fact, I hope it will be banned.

CHAPTER SEVENTEEN

ASSESSMENTS

Peals of laughter rang out in the spacious dining room that adjoined the open-plan kitchen. It was a Saturday morning. The radiance of young, fresh faces lit up the room. When friends of my daughters, Lauren and Rose came together to put the world to rights, the atmosphere was charged with their energy and enthusiasm, punctuated by squeals of delight. This was a joy to experience, in total contrast to the workplaces I occupied. What a privilege to be all students together!

Lauren was in the third year of her five-year course, training to be a vet, but the majority were in their second year of A Levels along with Rose, my younger daughter.

This scene, repeated most weeks is a treasured memory. Their good-humoured teasing often included me. One observed that I was 'not a proper parent.' Many of theirs wouldn't have allowed such a gathering. Well – as a single parent, I didn't know how to be one, did I? I made it up as I went along.

Nearly three years of full-time work, tests, essays, assessments and exams were behind me. The State Registered Final loomed, but before that I thought I'd record four of the assessments which stand out for different reasons.

The drug round. A qualified nurse checked my dispensing of medication to patients whilst a tutor observed. The tutor was Eric, a gentleman of large proportions who perspired visibly when stressed. At the start of our training, he'd demonstrated how to make a bed. Three handkerchiefs were drenched in the process!

Drugs, however were his speciality, so he had an air of confidence that day, evinced by his beaming smile and the twinkle in his eyes. More for his enjoyment of the subject than needing to assess my pharmaceutical knowledge, he grilled me for an hour afterwards. I passed.

What was sad about Eric was that he had a drink problem. His wife had left him; he lived in a house that was hospital accommodation. Eventually, he was suspended and dismissed, not long after I qualified.

Feeling shamed and betrayed, he soon became deeply depressed. I gave him emotional support on the phone for several months but it wasn't enough to stop him taking his life with a drugs overdose. It's sad to think that the help we were trained to provide was apparently not available to him. No one offered. He ended his life alone in his one-bedroomed flat within a town centre tower block. I'd worried that he hadn't answered the phone for over a week, but assumed he might have gone to stay with his son. The bad news travelled fast, once we learned what had happened because his son also worked as an RMN. It still saddens me to recall this event.

The second assessment was straight-forward, involving the recording of a patient's vital signs; BP, temperature, pulse and respirations. It would have been hard to fail that… although we had only one chance at getting it right, on one patient.

The third was a jolly affair, although the name doesn't describe it. Total Patient Care. Most female student nurses usually bathed a patient and did their hair. I don't know what the two male students did because they were on placement in a different hospital.

However, my choice of activity was to deliver a counselling session, based on *Transactional Analysis. The willing participant was the delightful patient with whom I had great accord once she'd begun to recover from a serious suicide attempt. It was Stella.

I introduced Stella to the theory of TA in front of a Charge Nurse who was assessing me. She was intrigued by the exercises which threw light on her decision-making processes as well as revelations about what informed her behaviour, according to TA. Much chortling ensued. Everyone seemed to enjoy it and I passed with flying colours. Sometime later, I learned that the Charge Nurse had known nothing about TA before the assessment. He'd had to give himself a crash course before becoming the examiner.

Being in charge of a ward for one day, was the final one. This was a boring ordeal. It concerned nothing in which I was interested. Overseeing the mundane routine of the day, like ensuring appointments and interviews took place; assigning staff their tasks; answering the phone; putting entries in the diary; managing altercations between patients and staff should they arise. It meant mostly being office-bound which I hated.

The words of our tutor in 'Introductory Block' came back to haunt me, causing a sinking feeling in the pit of my stomach:

'Don't think, as an RMN that you'll have time to talk to the patients. You'll be too busy running the ward.'

This, as I've said before, was the last thing I'd thought being a psychiatric nurse was about.

How, I'd wondered, could I make it more of what I'd hoped it would be? It was September 1988, when I sat and passed the final three-hour exam.

A few months later, I would undergo a major operation which, ultimately and paradoxically would help me realize the dream I had cherished – that of being a counsellor, whose job it was to talk to patients all day and every day.

Until then, being on a ward of nearly thirty patients was the only destiny on the horizon. It wasn't a prospect I relished, unlike my fellow students. They couldn't wait.

*Transactional Analysis was a theory developed by Eric Berne, a Canadian psychiatrist in the 1950-60s. It propounded the belief that self-understanding could be gained from analysing people's social interactions through conversations, particularly when they 'went wrong.'

TA can enable people to communicate better and be more effective in their lives. Best of all, they can learn to do it for themselves. They don't need an expert interpreter. It fitted well with my desire to help patients enable themselves.

I researched several different psychological interventions in my own time, because I still thought psychiatric nursing was about understanding people, their problems and most of all, empowering them to work their way through the difficulties life poses for us all.

CHAPTER EIGHTEEN

MORE ON Dr F

Wherever I went now, on a placement, Dr F's reputation seemed to gather momentum, if such a thing can happen. It was like a dark storm cloud, burgeoning on the horizon. The idea, as described in a previous chapter, that he could section patients as a punishment for the angry behaviour *he'd* provoked, didn't end there.

'He renews them. If he doesn't like someone and they're on a Section 3, he just finds excuses to keep them detained.' This was said more than once. On occasions, in the medium to long stay hospital, certain individuals were identified by staff, who had been subjected to this. Years of it.

Another story which circulated was about changing patients' notes, to suit his version of events, were he challenged. It would have been an easy thing to do because the medical notes were loose leaved and simply bound by cord in a folder, so any of them could have been replaced. I couldn't ascertain the truth of this at all, but a picture was emerging bit by bit, of a man who was the antithesis of the desirable characteristics hoped for, in a health care professional.

I suppose that families of the patients didn't question this, because he was the trusted expert, wasn't he? At that time, most people, including staff seemed to attribute consultants with a mysterious kind of power – believing them to have special knowledge which could diagnose what was wrong with people.

Years later, I realise that all they did, for the most part, was to categorise sets of symptoms (behaviours), label them as recognised 'disorders' (as per DSM III) and prescribe medication to reduce/eliminate the symptoms, without addressing the causes. What would be the point of that? If the symptoms were 'cured', then the problems would disappear, wouldn't they? As if by magic.

Sometimes I glimpsed him, at a distance. He was flashily dressed with an air of self-importance. Generally, he wore dark, fashionable suits but with brightly coloured shirts and no tie. He was softly spoken with a somewhat disguised, gentrified local accent. On one particular day, it wasn't for long. He'd gathered up his cronies and disappeared off the ward, at a time when his ward round was supposed to be taking place.

'Where's Dr F?' I'd innocently asked.

'Gone to the seaside' replied an SEN. 'It's what he does.'

To say that I was taken aback, would be an understatement. Doctors should have been meeting with, and interviewing their patients at this time, although, as I've said – very few actually did, to my knowledge.

'He does the ward round over the phone sometimes,' said another. This latter habit would have tragic consequences a few months after I'd left the profession, but for years, he got away with it.

'More of his patients commit suicide than any of the other "psychs" put together,' observed a female SEN who'd been around for years, adding swiftly, 'Off the ward. So, nothing to do with him. That's when he changes the notes.' This never seemed to be queried by anyone…

It was said that he had had a troubled background. Seen one of his siblings come to a tragic end; but I don't know how true that was. His wife was an English, female psychiatrist who also worked in the same establishments. They had four sons, apparently – three of whom were allegedly conceived, following reconciliations of their disrupted, dysfunctional relationship.

Dr F was reputed to have had several affairs with members of staff. At their final parting, a year or two later, I was told that he had tried to kidnap his sons, when she'd threatened to leave him, but his estranged wife had fled the country with their children and settled somewhere as far away as she could.

A curious quirk of hers had been remarked on by a staff nurse I worked with, when 'Care in the Community' began to be introduced. This involved patients' being given the chance for semi-independent living off the ward in some purpose-built houses that were within the hospital grounds.

'She has favourites' said the Staff Nurse, 'and Dora isn't one of them. That's why she keeps her on the ward and refuses to sign her out of here.'

Dora was a patient who repeated all day long that she 'wanted to go to her own home' and this accommodation, although not 'home' could have fulfilled part of what she longed for. Seems the couple had some things in common. An abuse of power.

One day, a Charge Nurse was enthusing about a 'new therapy' that Dr F was practising. RET (Rational Emotive Therapy by Albert Ellis).

Except that it wasn't. RET invites the sufferer to peel back their beliefs to question the disabling messages we sometimes give ourselves, when we are trying to attain a goal. Self-defeating statements in all their forms are challenged, then a reality check is suggested to test their veracity.

Dr F's was a short form version, although I'm being charitable here. The Charge Nurse explained that you just have to ask 'Why?' to everything a patient utters. The distress and despair that this could invoke in someone who is emotionally disturbed is unimaginable.

However, undesirable behaviours that resulted and may in fact have been a normal, angry reaction to this kind of provocation (being asked why all the time), were often ascribed to the patient's ongoing 'disorder'. This is what happened with 'Disinhibited Dorothy', who told Dr S exactly what she thought of him, when he came across her and asked her how she was.

I didn't realize at the time, that after qualifying, I would witness Dr F's inaccurate practice of RET in action; object strongly to the effect it had on one of my clients, in the Day Hospital and ultimately, have conditions of work imposed on me, that I couldn't tolerate, so as to be felt forced to leave.

Looking back some thirty-five years later, it's hard to believe that such malpractice was witnessed and tolerated.

At best, people seemed to view him as 'a bit of a character' whilst others were disturbed, but too fearful to speak out against a powerful psychiatrist. Staff mostly muttered about him in the background.

How many women have been incarcerated for having strong views which defied the status quo? It's happened down the ages, right up to present day. Sadly, it will probably carry on.

SHUT UP AND KEEP TAKING THE PILLS

CHAPTER NINETEEN

PARADOX

Many years earlier, the Flying Squad Ambulance Service came to rescue me from a home labour which had gone drastically wrong. At one point during the thirty-six-hour ordeal, my then husband had to sign a form authorizing the medics to preserve my life rather than the baby's.

Thankfully, Lauren was born, but the exhaustion and trauma heralded a protracted period of post-natal depression that probably contributed to the breakdown of the couple relationship. Antidepressants and tranquillisers did nothing to restore it. Just rendered me almost incapable of functioning, beyond seeing to my little one's needs.

At the time, I didn't question the GP's prescribing this medication. It's with hindsight and being made more aware of the adverse effects on patients that I realise how badly the psychoactive drugs affected me. All those years ago, they were prescribed in much higher doses than in the 1980s.

Twenty years earlier, it was believed that they were the new wonder cure for depression and anxiety. By the evenings, I had a pounding headache that barely allowed me to lean over my baby, to change her. It must have been the drugs, but side effects were never discussed nor mentioned! The headache was most likely thought to be part of the depression.

During the first few months of qualifying as an RMN, period pain intensified. Fibroids were the cause. For two days in every menstrual cycle, my body was convulsed in agonizing relentless torment, accompanied by the need to change protection every two hours. This time, a major operation was necessary.

The only solution was to have a hysterectomy, so several painful months later, it was scheduled and then performed accordingly, in June 1989.

Neither the severe distress of my first labour nor the extremely painful periods in later life could have prepared me for the level of suffering I endured in the Recovery Room some while after the operation. It was indescribable.

Never a patient patient, I began to bawl at the top of my voice, 'Help! I want some painkillers and I want them **now**!' The momentary in-breath of air needed to fill my lungs, gave me temporary slight relief from feeling that my insides had been ripped out with a rusty knife.

I must have repeated this plea twenty times or more before a young registrar approached me and said, 'Hazel. Your blood pressure's too low. We can't give you anymore just now.' He began to walk away. Summoning all my strength, I grabbed the sleeve of his smart suit and heard the stitches ripping as I wrenched it from his arm, still bellowing with even greater vigour, 'I want painkillers and I want them **NOW**!!'

They must have given me something after that, because I remembered nothing more until the middle of the night when a firm hospital bed on a ward afforded me minimal comfort.

Not for long, however, because the agony started all over again. The clock dictated when injections of Omnipon were due, but the relief it gave was short-lived. When I could eventually read my drugs chart, I discovered that Paracetamol was on offer and – miracle of miracles, this worked better than the controlled drug!

Once discharged from hospital, there were twelve weeks during which to recover. This was greatly helped by my elderly Mum who had come to live with me, the year before and my kind fiancé who did the same, at a time of great need.

By October, however, it was obvious that working on the ward I'd previously been assigned to, was out of the question. Heavy lifting would be involved. Following a hysterectomy, lifting nothing heavier than a bag of sugar was advised for the first six weeks. Was my nursing career at an end?

I knew nothing about the Day Hospital at that time, but suddenly I learned there was a vacancy for a member of staff to work there. Imagine my delight when I also learned that this work was counselling Outpatients. No more lifting, bathing, bodily fluids, tending wounds… controlling my excitement when I interviewed for this post was the main challenge.

Success! It seemed (for a while) to be my pinnacle of joy. It was what I'd always thought Psychiatric Nursing was about. Talking to people; hearing their stories; helping them through emotional traumas; discovering together, ways in which they could help them help themselves.

Psychiatrists referred patients for counselling. I've already mentioned that psychiatrists rarely made an appearance outside of their offices. They saw patients behind closed doors in clinics and sometimes talked about them with a chosen few staff in a weekly ward round – also behind closed doors.

In the Day Hospital, here, psychiatrists were never seen. Referrals were made by letter. At daily morning meetings, we volunteered to engage with individuals whom we believed we could help.

One fateful day, I volunteered to work with a patient of Dr F's. For a few months, all would be well, as I delighted in giving the service which enabled people to live their lives to the full.

Unfortunately, the big black cloud that was Dr F became the factor that engineered my downfall and, as I'll describe, Dr F became responsible for ending my short yet successful career in the profession.

CHAPTER TWENTY

BREATHING FREE

It might seem curious that one sunny afternoon in October, I could be seen, standing still, with one foot on a piece of desiccated white dog poo. My companion, Martha, a woman in her forties, who had put on one of her best frocks for the occasion, composed herself and after a few moments' hesitation, followed suit.

Perhaps it's hard to believe that this was part of the work of the Cognitive Behavioural Psychotherapy Department, but they dealt with phobias of all descriptions. This one was very common, as were fear of public toilets, fear of dogs, fear of going out, to name but a few.

The antidote to this was very simple. The theory was that it wasn't possible to maintain a state of heightened anxiety (rated 10). In a state of fear, we most often hyperventilate. Patients were taught to control their breathing – gradually reducing the rhythm down to what was normal for them, whilst at the same time noticing the reduction in their discomfort, verbalising the reducing numbers as this took place.

SHUT UP AND KEEP TAKING THE PILLS

Martha began the exercise which by now, after much practice, was second nature. The 'best frock' also gave her confidence. I watched her shoulders, raised at first (fight or flight syndrome) and had the happy satisfaction of hearing her slowly count down to 2, at which point she followed my lead.

This placement was beyond what should have been the end of my training. I'd missed six weeks of the three-year course when a road traffic accident which I've written about elsewhere, resulted in hospitalisation and had caused me to have delayed concussion. The number of weeks lost recuperating from this event had to be made up, so I was the only student to experience the joys of the CBT Department.

CBT specialists were paid considerably more than qualified nurses to perform this therapy. Bit of a rarefied atmosphere! Although CBT was a specialism, the department had the same shabby décor as the rest of the psychiatric department. Magnolia-painted walls hung with uninteresting pictures; the furniture was worn and the floors hard.

There were two offices for the respective psychotherapists. Simon was Ellen's senior, so he had a noticeably larger one and then each had a cubby hole of a therapy room in which they received patients. Both were heavy smokers – but not in front of the patients!

The two specialists were complete opposites. Simon was dour, almost monosyllabic, and tall, with a ginger beard. Ellen was twinkly, energized, and Scottish. My placement attached me to Ellen. We laughed a lot together but the work was serious. It had the power to change people's lives.

Toilets and dog poo were a bit depressing. I'd got used to being given 'funny looks' in the ladies, although it didn't help that this was an area in which we didn't wear uniform.

SHUT UP AND KEEP TAKING THE PILLS

Several unsuspecting members of the general public would come upon two women standing stock still outside a cubicle; the one smiling with encouragement towards the other who would be somewhat slowly and inexplicably to outsiders, voicing random numbers and visibly focussing on her breathing. This procedure would be repeated as many times as were necessary in stages, towards the most feared object of all – the toilet seat.

At its conclusion, there would be congratulations and triumphal gasps. Some of the public must have reported it to others as if witnessing a surreal and mystifying event. The less charitable would have probably dismissed us both as 'mad.'

The treatment wasn't as noticeable when I worked outside. Indeed, this is what I liked best: travelling on local buses with people who were agoraphobic. It was a delight to enable them to come out of their self-imprisoned world and share the sights and sounds of the great outdoors.

John hadn't left home for the previous ten years, following a traumatic incident at his place of work. It was towards the end of my six-week placement that he plucked up courage to venture out with me, all the while focussing on his breathing and noting the reducing numbers. Once on the bus, it was a revelation for him to see how the local landscape had changed.

It's like a different world,' he said, with his hands excitedly gripping the seat in front. There were cries of: 'Blummin' 'eck! Wot were that?' and 'Where's that gone?' as he witnessed the fact that some landmarks he'd once known had disappeared, to be replaced by others. It was gratifying that his interest in external surroundings nullified his fears of being out.

Something as ordinary as getting on a bus had transformed him. He returned uplifted, excited, and eager to go again. Seeing people released from their respective phobias was uplifting for me, too. The lives of those who were suffering were enhanced and restored.

Ellen and I both rejoiced when patients conquered their fears and began, sometimes for the first time in years, to lead a normal life. I felt privileged to play a small part in this. Something remarkable came out of the accident I'd had. It also gave me several weeks' free time to be able to begin to organize my life in a new home!

CHAPTER TWENTY-ONE

THE BEGINNING OF THE END

1989 saw my distressing ordeal of physical pain brought to an end.

1990 seemed to fulfil all my hopes and dreams. I married for the second time, after twenty years alone and we spent an idyllic honeymoon abroad, over the following two weeks.

By July, Lauren graduated as a vet. Rose gained a double first in biology and geology, carrying on to achieve a first, as well, in another three years it took her to do a doctorate, following the first degree course she completed.

The hysterectomy from which I'd now recovered gave me the opportunity to work in the way I did best, at the Day Hospital. The case-load numbered twenty and most clients benefitted greatly from the counselling. *This* is what I'd thought psychiatry was about.

My mission was to keep people out of the Psychiatric Hospital, off the mind-numbing drugs and equally importantly, without having to have labels for the symptoms which pathologized their normal reactions to abnormal events. Very often, I didn't read the psychiatrist's referral because it would have labels which masked the underlying stories of what had happened to someone.

Carla sparked my interest. In the morning meeting when referrals were allocated, I volunteered to see her. In this case, I couldn't help but notice that at age, 24, she was said to have 'endogenous depression.'

'Reactive' and 'Endogenous' depression were terms used in those days. Essentially, it meant that the cause or causes for 'reactive' depression were obvious; less so for endogenous. The latter implied an illness that had been long term. This intrigued me because of her age. She was so young. It was possible that traumatic events in her life may, as yet unspoken, have contributed to this diagnosis. Without realizing that this was a patient of Dr F's, at the time, I declared I'd be glad to see her.

Carla was small in stature. Her clothes seemed to envelop her, almost hiding her diminutive frame. She had a habit of clutching them around her as she sat in the chair. Quietly spoken; sometimes hesitating between words, as if she dare not risk voicing them. She was difficult to get to know. Very guarded in what she said. The weekly sessions brought about painfully slow progress although trust between us began to be established.

Family relationship problems were hinted at, but she had a habit of giving a little bit of information and then clamming up. The sessions at this time were unlimited, so clients could go at their own pace.

Some years later, working for EAPs as a freelance counsellor where as few as five or six sessions were the norm, I had to learn to work more swiftly. Carla must have had about twelve over a three-month period, before she began to talk about the abuse she'd suffered in the past. Then, after a while, her mood plummeted to an all-time low. She began to talk of feeling suicidal and I feared for her safety.

As Carla began to reveal events from her past, she experienced a sense of shame that was becoming overwhelming.

'I don't deserve to live,' was a phrase repeated all too often, accompanied by the clutching of her clothes, as if she wanted to make herself disappear.

I worked hard to steer her away from this view and for a time, it seemed to work until one day, she said, 'I know what I'm going to do.' Her young face was set in determined lines.

I asked her to tell me.

'I'll take all my tablets,' she replied, simply.

Nothing I said following this carried any weight against her tragic resolve, so somewhat in desperation, rather than in hope, I persuaded her to see her psychiatrist, Dr F.

It was only the second time in my short 5-year career that I thought of seeking the help of a psychiatrist. Carla's intentions were to be taken seriously. She had a plan. I hoped that the psychiatrist would show empathy and compassion. She agreed to do so, providing I accompanied her.

On the fateful day, Dr F couldn't have looked more unconcerned if he'd tried. He was seated at an angle to the desk with his feet resting on it. Barely looking up when we entered, he waved a hand towards two chairs placed *behind* it. We felt disadvantaged from the start. Carla disappeared into a low club chair that scarcely allowed her to be seen above his desk and I had an upright one which made me feel awkward.

Every room in the counselling area of the Day Hospital had chairs that matched one another in terms of their height, size, and comfort – so important it is, to establish the equality of the participants.

There was no greeting. No welcome. He picked up a paper from his desk, presumably to remind himself whom he had in front of him and scowled at the name. The tone of the meeting was set by his first few words, 'So, you think you are a shitty person? Why?'

Although this would be considered to be mild swearing by today's standards, it was absolutely forbidden in those days, for any member of staff to speak in this way to a patient. As I've mentioned before, this was Dr F's way of conducting RET. Another forbidden word in *counselling* is 'Why?' It is too accusatory and implies blame or judgment on the part of the counsellor.

Dr F got away with this, because he was a law unto himself. He was 'the expert in RET' in this part of the hospital. It was most unlike the CBT that was practised in the Cognitive Behavioural Psychotherapy Department where I'd worked with Simon and Ellen.

Nurses knew little about these relatively new ways of working. No one questioned *his* methods, which is why I came to be punished eventually, for speaking out.

For reasons of confidentiality, I cannot detail the content of this confrontation. Suffice to say that with almost every utterance of Dr F's, Carla shrivelled further into the chair. She was bombarded with questions, peppered with implied insults, and constantly asked 'Why?'

I could see that her eyes were welling with tears. Finally, he refused to help her. He claimed that she wasn't serious in her threat to kill herself. He wasn't convinced. I was torn between wanting to argue her case, or getting her to a place of safety. The latter won, in the end because Dr F was immutable and from his animated demeanour was clearly enjoying the effect he was having on Carla. Here was first hand evidence of all the rumours I'd overheard about his attitude to patients. Cruel and arrogant. Abusing his power.

SHUT UP AND KEEP TAKING THE PILLS

My embarrassment and extreme disappointment were only suppressed by my need to comfort Carla. She was almost hysterical, saying over and over, when we'd left the room that she'd never felt like killing herself more than after meeting him. It took two hours of comforting, soothing and reassuring her. She was still overwrought, however so I took the drastic step of escorting her to A&E. I stayed with her, until I was certain that she would be admitted, before I could go home, by which time it was quite late in the evening.

The next morning, I discovered that of course, Dr F was furious that I had 'gone over his head.' Looking back, it's obvious that he set out to punish us both and show who was 'Boss.' He had had Carla re-admitted to another hospital that was miles away from the Day Hospital.

This was obviously an attempt to ensure that I couldn't see her. Despite that, I made the effort to visit her, to assure her that I hadn't been party to this transfer. My hopes of maintaining the trusting relationship I had so painstakingly built up were further dashed, when I arrived.

The Nurse in charge of the ward was the very same crony of Dr F's who had laughed with glee some months earlier, when he was reporting how F practised this new therapy of RET, consisting of asking 'Why' over and over again.

We met in a side room. Carla was in a dreadful state. She spluttered with anger about Dr F's treatment of her. Her face was bright red and contorted. Her manner was loud and threatening. Although her wrath was fully justified, the Charge Nurse overheard the commotion from the other side of the door; stormed in with another nurse in tow and Carla was carted off to be given a shot of diazepam.

A day or two, later, I learned that he'd misinterpreted the situation and reported that I had visited her and distressed her. I feel sure

Carla would have told him it was because of the meeting with Dr F, but as I've said – the Charge Nurse was a crony. He distorted the truth, to cover for his friend.

When I wrote up the notes later, to be able to establish the real truth of events, my fate was sealed. The following day, I was on annual leave for two weeks. It was one of the unhappiest holidays I've ever had.

When I returned to work, The Nursing Officer called me into the office. 'You're suspended, Hazel, pending an enquiry,' he announced with a degree of shame, I thought.

Everyone knew Dr F's practices were suspect but no one would stand up against him, nor speak out. The Sister who was in charge of the Day Hospital, frog-marched me through all the hospital corridors to the front door, and told me: '*On no account, must you talk to anyone from work.*'

I left; walking the long, straight road to my home, with a growing sense of isolation, despair and desperation.

CHAPTER TWENTY-TWO

TRANSGRESSION

How tender is the intimacy of kind words
balm to the soul
they can heal the pain of harm
that caused a heart to break
the assaulted spirit is replenished
re-invigorated with a will
to live
to love.
Restored

We were drilled throughout our 3 years' training: '*Always* put the patient first!'

Sacrosanct, or so we were led to believe until, as it turned out, you witnessed a psychiatrist abusing his power, to the detriment of a vulnerable human being he was supposed to be helping. He knew best, though, didn't he? You didn't question that.

Except, I did. Not just question it, but dared to criticize him as well. Unwisely, in the patient's records, written up just before annual leave, I suggested that Dr F had used the patient like some sort of pawn in a power game (when he moved her to a hospital far away), causing her to feel isolated and abandoned.

We were a multidisciplinary team so my notes about events were available for others to read.

The special relationship of client and counsellor wasn't widely understood at that time. My supervision partner, Sybil referred to counselling as 'a piece of piss', meaning that it was an easy, not very important thing to do. I strongly disliked that remark. The initial dependency on the counsellor is necessary for the client's growth in order to provide a corrective emotional experience. This engenders mutual trust and through that, the client learns to trust him or herself which accelerates self-healing.

It began to dawn on me that this early stage of counselling was being misinterpreted as being 'overly involved.' What ensued in the case of Carla was unforgiveable on my part, because the patient trusted me more than the psychiatrist!

At one point, during the time I was waiting to attend the disciplinary, I was sent to Occupational Health to have my mental state assessed. The inference was that I must be mad to have gone against a psychiatrist. They at least had the good grace to find out that there was nothing wrong with me. No mental instability of any kind.

If I'd had nightmares during my two weeks' annual leave, about being forced to abandon Carla or possibly lose my job for gross misconduct, they were as nothing compared with the pain I endured during the weeks before the disciplinary. This was made far worse by the Union Rep who was hardly ever there, when I phoned. She was:

SHUT UP AND KEEP TAKING THE PILLS

Unavailable
In a meeting
Off sick
On annual leave

Or she 'would phone me back' (which she never did).

The longest conversation we had, was half an hour before the hearing took place, six weeks after the suspension.

'It's looking very bad for you, Hazel. You could be sacked for this. It could be construed as gross misconduct.'

My protests fell on deaf ears, even with her. No one would believe that Dr F had been the one to upset Carla. The focus was entirely on me for this apparent wrong-doing.

Being banned from speaking to anyone at work, did me no favours at all. I thought my supervision partner, Sybil could give me the support I needed. She was ten years my senior and had been in the NHS for several decades. She, amongst others had recounted damning stories about Dr F. So, I took a big risk and rang her to ask for her support as a witness to his misbehaviours. How naïve. She promised she would, but the night before the hearing, I discovered a message on the answerphone. She declined to appear. She was afraid for her job. I had to assume that, because we never spoke again.

'Don't say anything at all, Hazel. Leave it to me. It could be the worse for you, if you speak,' cautioned the Union Rep as we met for the afore-mentioned half hour, ahead of the hearing. This was once she'd listened to my version of events. There wasn't time to reason with her or ask why. Whose side was she on?

That became clear when we presented ourselves in the dark, cavernous room that was the Chief Nursing Officer's office. She laboured the point about my inexperience.

'A very young nurse,' she proclaimed in shrill tones that echoed through the room.

'Perhaps not in years,' said with a smirk, 'but in all other respects, she has a lot to learn.'

The Nursing Officer nodded and kept silent as she droned on in this vein, for another ten minutes or so. Then it was all over. He scraped his chair backwards, barely suppressing a yawn, rose to his feet and stared impassively at me.

'We'll let you know our decision in the next two weeks, Nurse Jones,' and with that he disappeared into another room.

I'd been silenced, like the patients – except without medication. The Union Rep had effectively told me to hold my tongue.

Over the next two weeks, I had sleepless nights and lost my appetite. Angry thoughts about the injustice of it, not least the peremptory way in which it had been handled, vied with the grief I felt for all the clients I'd be forced to abandon if I lost my job. How would they feel and react when someone to whom they'd opened their hearts, had suddenly vanished without explanation? I felt bereft. Powerless.

When the letterbox snapped open, as it delivered the verdict, my stomach lurched with anxiety. Thereafter, I always experienced this sensation when mail was delivered on a Saturday. Communications about my case came without exception, at the weekend when I could do nothing about them, thereby causing the most extreme distress.

SHUT UP AND KEEP TAKING THE PILLS

This letter informed me of three things:

1) My relationship with the patient had been inappropriate.

2) I was 'overly involved.'

3) I would be moved immediately, back to the ward I'd worked on previously, and be under the supervision of Dr F's wife.

Impossible. This resolution was untenable, not least because of having close contact with F's wife. Was this a deliberate ploy to force me to leave? But the Union Rep warned me not to appeal, 'Or it could be worse.' The soul searching was agonizing, although ultimately, I felt I had no choice but to resign.

When I contacted them for advice, the Royal College of Nursing said it was constructive dismissal and suggested I file a complaint. I duly did so. They took three long years to decide it wasn't worth pursuing. Meanwhile, one day when I was shopping in the market, I discovered that a former patient had been told that I'd died. This had allegedly been said by the Sister who'd frog-marched me off the premises.

My disillusionment with psychiatry was complete or rather, with some of the staff, who practised it in such a perfidious way.

Dr F could have been stopped in his tracks if others had come forward and supported me. How many patients had he harmed in his career and not been apprehended? Well, eventually, he was. The circumstances were so very sad, and maybe if people had listened to what I could have told them, a death could have been avoided. I'll write about that in another chapter.

CHAPTER TWENTY- THREE

TRAGEDY

Only 5 months after my resignation, shocking news hit the headlines. It was soon picked up by the national papers, too. An 11-year-old girl had died in the town's shopping centre, stabbed to death by a female psychiatric patient. The perpetrator's psychiatrist was Dr F.

The story that unfolded was heart-breaking, tragic but worst of all – predictable. Infamous for his arrogance, Dr F had gone against not only the advice of nursing staff who'd warned she was dangerous, but also the decision of a Mental Health Tribunal who'd voted against releasing this patient. Dr F ignored them all; discharged her, on the grounds that she'd probably do something bad which would incur a longer detention.

She had threatened she 'would kill someone' and by this time had already attacked another patient on the ward, before he ordered her discharge over the 'phone from his home. He didn't even attend the ward to assess her in person.

The news was devastating. I'd effectively committed professional suicide when I'd tried to say his practice was unsafe because I'd witnessed his provoking behaviour towards Carla. She'd said she 'wanted to kill herself more than at any other time in her life, after meeting him.' He'd made her feel worthless.

No one had listened to me. Other witnesses to his unprofessional manner were too cowardly to come forward. This latest tragedy might have been prevented. The little girl's life might have been saved. I wept for the parents.

Dr A had retired just as I was about to undergo the disciplinary, but I phoned him at home to talk about the sad events. He was sympathetic, but what he said was surprising.

'We tried, Hazel.' He named another psychiatrist. 'We tried to warn people about his dubious behaviours and we met with the same kind of opposition.' I expressed dismay and wondered out loud how this could be. He had no explanation but went on to say, 'When there's an enquiry, you can be sure that we'll give the evidence of what we know.'

Despite events, Dr F continued to practise at the same hospital for several months. An internal enquiry by those with vested interests, appeared to allow this to happen. A local MP, however, had other ideas.

In a speech he delivered to the House of Commons, he called for a Public Enquiry. Of course, it took several months to be convened, but at least it was thorough. Dr F was found guilty of multiple charges of negligence.

He was ordered to re-train for six months outside of the local area, but allowed back to practise in a senior role at the same hospital, albeit under supervision, once he'd completed retraining. He should have been sacked and prevented from working ever again.

There were repercussions for him in his private life. Villagers where he lived drove him out of his home. The pictures of this are still in the public domain, too. His former house stands, wrecked and abandoned with several classic cars left to rot in the garages and a swimming pool taken over by weeds. Dr A informed me that his wife had left him and taken their sons to live abroad. It's amazing that he had the temerity to go back to work in the same place, but perhaps no one else in their right minds would have employed him.

There was another murder by stabbing, twenty years later in a local park. The victim was a teenaged girl and the female relative of someone I know. Circumstances were similar. A female psychiatric patient who had threatened to kill someone. She wasn't safe to be on the streets, yet she had been released. I don't know who her psychiatrist was.

I was left feeling vindicated but very troubled. The MP who facilitated a Public Enquiry about the murder of the little girl said I should ask for a judicial review of my case. It seemed pointless. It wouldn't bring the little girl back and why would I want to work in such a toxic environment?

I thought I'd heard and seen the last of Dr F, but I was wrong. There would be a time even after I'd moved to another town, when his venomous influence would be felt by me. More of that another time?

POST SCRIPT

I never lost my belief in the power of counselling to change lives.

It would take me another five years before I achieved the status of a freelance counsellor. There were many setbacks along the way.

However, I can now look back over more than thirty-five years of having had the honour and privilege of playing a small but significant part in hundreds of people's lives.

ODE TO A COUNSELLOR

Have you the time to share my pain
a little of the agony?
Bereft, defenceless, worn with care
I sit before you, soul laid bare
and beg you make me whole again

Don't turn, don't spurn me
spend a while
and listen to my tortuous grief
I need acceptance and relief
from thoughts that weigh so heavily

The care you give me now can call
me back from black despair and death
Don't underestimate your power
to change my life and keep me safe

Befriend, defend me, help me cope
tho' time you may not want to give
This hour I could discover hope
and strength to find the will to live

In saving me, you save yourself
Who knows when roles reverse, you may
need me to comfort and support you
push the doubts and fears away

SHUT UP AND KEEP TAKING THE PILLS

So spend a while and hear me when
the time you may not want to spare.
Caring, sharing fellow feeling
unburdens me, begins the healing
makes me want to live again

HIERARCHY OF STAFF IN MENTAL ILLNESS NURSING 1985-1991

SENIOR NURSING OFFICER
DEPUTY NURSING OFFICER
CHARGE NURSE OR SISTER
(of equal status)

SENIOR STAFF NURSE (Male or female)
The above were formerly Deputy Charge Nurse and Deputy Sister
which identified their respective genders

STAFF NURSE

STATE ENROLLED NURSE

NURSING CARE ASSISTANT

STUDENT NURSE

*Rather curiously, for many years a 'Matron' was female, but in this century, a Matron can also be male. The youngest student in our intake eventually went on to become Matron over all the Wards in the long stay hospital. Quite an exalted position.

BIOGRAPHY

Hazel Jones has been a freelance counsellor for many years. Her first husband deserted the family and left them homeless. This brought her into contact with the psychiatric services, initially as a patient (with a broken heart). It was then that she met Dr A after which she believed that psychiatry was about talking to people to help them cope with life. Such adverse circumstances were eventually faced with courage and fortitude, but there were many other hurdles to overcome, until she realised the dream of becoming a counsellor who helped others to help themselves. This book describes one of those many episodes. Perhaps there could be other books in the future.

Printed in Great Britain
by Amazon

28486524R00066